Significant Event Audit

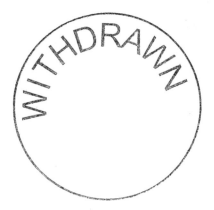

Significant Event Audit

A focus for clinical governance

Jonathan Stead

and

Grace Sweeney

Kingsham

First published 2001
by Kingsham Press

Oldbury Complex
Marsh Lane
Easthampnett
Chichester, West Sussex
PO18 OJW
United Kingdom

Typeset in AGaramond

Printed and bound by
MPG Books
Bodmin
Cornwall
United Kingdom

53616

W
84.3
STE

ISBN: 1-904235-00-X

British Library Cataloging in Publication Data
A catalogue record of this book is available from the British Library

Stead, Jonathan & Sweeney, Grace

About the authors

Dr. Jonathan Stead MPhil., MBBS, MRCGP
Jonathan Stead has worked as a General Practitioner in a small dispensing practice, north of Exeter, since 1980. He has been Chairman of the Primary Care Audit Group in North and East Devon since its inception. He is also a Research Fellow at the Research and Development Support Unit at the University of Exeter. His particular interests are in quality improvement, learning from experience (Significant Event Audit) and the organisational aspects of care for people with diabetes and asthma.

He has worked with Dr. Grace Sweeney and Dr. Richard Westcott for three years, researching the benefits of SEA. He has been involved at both regional and national level with education and facilitation to introduce and sustain SEA in variety of settings, ranging from primary and secondary health care to social care and prison health care.

Dr. Grace Sweeney PhD., MPhil., DipCot.
Grace Sweeney trained as an occupational therapist in Dublin in the early 1980s, after which she spent several years working in the field of acute and adult mental health. During her time as a clinician, she developed an interest in the ways in which health professionals – particularly those working with damaged and vulnerable people, protected themselves and their colleagues, whilst remaining open to pain and the distress of others. This interest was followed up by postgraduate studies for an MPhil. and PhD at the University of Exeter.

Her immediate post-doctoral work centred around the exploration of Significant Event Audit in primary care, secondary care and prison health care with Dr. Jonathan Stead and Dr. Richard Westcott. Grace is currently the South West's Research Fellow in Primary Care Clinical Governance, on a study which is exploring the development of clinical governance in primary care.

Acknowledgements

The development of Significant Event Audit in the emerging world of clinical governance would not have been possible without the enthusiasm, support and wisdom of our friend Richard Westcott.

Mary Fox was the lead researcher in the prison study and Rachel Perkin has been involved in workshops looking at sustaining the process of SEA.

This book was borne out of an idea floated at a one-day workshop held at St Thomas's Hospital in London on the 9th February 2000, which focused on the potential of SEA and future areas of research. The authors are grateful for the helpful contribution of the workshop attendees:

Professor Mike Pringle
Dr Richard Westcott
Mrs Mary Fox
Miss Liz Cosford
Dr Roger Pietroni
Dr Anita Berlin
Professor Jim Parle
Dr Steve Rogers
Dr Louise Robinson

The authors extend a special thanks to all the individuals who so willingly contributed to the research projects in a variety of health care settings.

Contents

Foreword

by Professor Mike Pringle, Chairman, Royal College of General Practitioners

Nobody does their job perfectly and no system of care gives ideal outcomes. We need to recognise and remember the continuum of quality, from poor care to "best" care that in reality means "better than the average". Everybody can improve; some need to improve more than others.

If clinical governance is to be effective in improving care for all people who use the health service, it must have tools that engage clinicians, managers, and teams at all points on the continuum. There will be many tools, including monitoring and feedback, conventional auditing, academic detailing, continuing professional development and risk management.

One methodology is emerging as being effective in many teams and in uniting all the disparate elements of clinical governance – significant event auditing. It includes all team members – doctors, nurses, managers, allied health professionals and receptionists – in the pursuit of quality. It is non-judgemental, but rigorous. It works with the existing culture. And most importantly is enjoyable.

The real strength of significant event auditing lies in harnessing the emotional content of cases, through a structured process, to achieve real changes. In my general practice we regularly audited the number of people with diabetes who had had their retina examined in the past year. The numbers hung around the 50% mark year after year and at each audit discussion we vowed to do better. When we discussed the case of an elderly woman living alone who had been diagnosed with advanced diabetic retinopathy, it all came to life for us. The commitment to retinal screening was hugely enhanced.

Those teams that have not taken up significant event auditing, and those primary care groups or trusts that are not encouraging it, need practical guidance. This book is exactly the guidance they seek. It explains the background, evidence and context. And it gives practical support to those interested in establishing it where they work.

If clinical governance is to support good care, identify excellence and encourage a climate of reflection and quality enhancement, then significant event auditing must be part of the activities of all teams. The concept and its application, as set out in this book, should become an ingrained part of our culture.

Professor Mike Pringle
2001

Part 1

Chapter 1

The context of Significant Event Audit

Dud: So would you say you've learned from your mistakes?
Pete: Oh yes, I'm sure I could repeat them exactly.

Peter Cook quoted by Brian Eno in *The Diary of Brian Eno*,
London: Faber & Faber, 1996.

1   WHAT IS SIGNIFICANT EVENT AUDIT?

Significant Event Audit (SEA) is a way to improve the quality of patient care. At a regular inter-professional team meeting, team members focus on particular incidents considered significant, to learn and improve from. More formally, it may be defined as:

> a process in which individual episodes, (when there has been a significant occurrence either beneficial or deleterious) are analysed, in a systematic and detailed way to ascertain what can be learnt about the overall quality of care, and to indicate changes that might lead to future improvements.
>
> after Pringle, 1995

2   SOME KEY CHARACTERISTICS

- SEA provides a systematic approach for teams to learn from experiences, both good and bad, in order to improve the quality of patient care. At a time of increasing complexity in healthcare, more care is delivered by inter-professional teams. These teams are usually from one organisation, or may straddle the interface between primary and secondary healthcare, or between health and social care.

- Communications between professional groups have long been a source of errors, while the interface between organisations is fraught with potential perils for the patient and their family.

- The regular SEA meeting acknowledges that errors will happen. The crucial issue is the response to the significant event. The traditional approach has been that mistakes did not happen (brushing them under the carpet) or to blame someone (never the senior team members).

- SEA meetings provide an opportunity to discuss improving systems of care, rather than making a member of the team a scapegoat. But the process of developing a team which trusts each other when discussing issues of extreme sensitivity takes time. These trusting teams emerge over months and years, needing careful support and leadership, as well as protected time to reflect. When healthcare organisations are being overwhelmed by increasing demand, is SEA a luxury which gets relegated to the status of 'it would be nice, if only we had the time'? It is at these times of increased pressure that errors occur, making it even more important that safe systems are in place.

- We believe that the investment of one hour a month (the golden hour) in SEA is repaid many times over. It has the potential for enabling safer systems, a learning environment, a stronger team and a caring group of professionals who are looking out for each other. As a consequence, it can enhance the quality of care provided by multi-professional teams. Additionally, it can minimize the likelihood of litigation and accompanying costs.

- It is important to emphasise that SEA is not just a reaction to an adverse event. It is an ongoing process, into which events, both good and not so good, are fed on a regular basis, to lead to a team approach to improving systems. If used as a knee-jerk response to an issue of poor performance, it will lead to serious damage to the team. SEA should come with a warning that stresses the importance of following some basic rules (more of this in Chapter 2).

Keeping to these simple rules can lead to impressive benefits in terms of improvements in the delivery of healthcare.

3   CLINICAL GOVERNANCE

A First Class Service: Quality in the New NHS was published in June 1998, setting out the concept of clinical governance. From April 1999, systems for the implementation of clinical governance began to emerge, including clear lines of accountability and accountability for the overall level of clinical care in health care organisations. Many of the building blocks, which together make up clinical governance, were already in existence, including clinical audit, research, evidence based practice, continuing professional development and issues relating to poor performance and complaints. The new idea was the interconnections between the blocks. For the first time, each organisation was encouraged to have a framework showing the relationships between activities which lead to quality improvement.

For Trusts, the introduction of clinical governance requires the chief executive to be the accountable person for quality, and therefore of similar importance to corporate governance. For the first time, quality featured at board meetings, and clinical governance sub-committees were

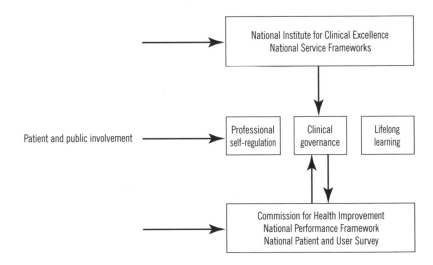

Adapted from *A First Class Service: Quality in the New NHS*

Figure 1. Setting, delivering and monitoring standards

set up to bring together the quality functions which had hitherto been run in isolation.

In general practice, the introduction of clinical governance presented challenges, since there was an under-developed approach to issues like risk management and human resources.

A number of well publicised medical errors, some repeated over a number of years, prompted the Chief Medical Officer, Professor Liam Donaldson, to publish a discussion document *An Organization with a Memory* in 2000. This paper developed the theme of learning from error and adverse incidents, as developed by the airline industry over the last thirty years, as well as work in the United States looking at harm caused to patients as a result of hospitalisation. In order to develop a culture which welcomes incident reporting rather than hiding it, a massive change is required by health care organisations, particularly against a backdrop of political spin and media frenzy.

Although the introduction of clinical governance in general practice required the development of a number of new support systems, there was one jewel whose time had come, especially as a means to develop an open, sharing, team approach to errors. This was **Significant Event Audit**. Throughout the United Kingdom there were pockets of enthusiasm for this approach, probably as a result of the pioneering work of Professor Mike Pringle, culminating in the publication of *Significant Event Auditing: a study of the feasibility and potential of case-based auditing in primary health care*. His approach was disseminated through a series of regional workshops, which equipped local leaders to spread the message about this powerful improvement tool.

The legacy of his work is an approach which allows primary health care teams to discuss events, both good and not so good, in a supportive inter-professional and dynamic way, soundly linked to individual and team learning.

Experience in other health and social care settings indicates that benefits can be accrued wherever patient care is delivered by inter-professional teams. The benefits of shared learning and openness seem to be universal, as long as some simple rules are followed. Breaking these rules can lead to a team catastrophe.

Chapter 2
Getting started – some simple rules

1 WHERE DO I BEGIN?

It is hard to get going with Significant Event Audit without external assistance. The good news is that there is plenty of help available. The skills required usually reside with clinical governance leads, clinical audit departments and clinical tutors. What they offer is some knowledge about the process of SEA, some facilitation and support for the team leader. They can guide you through the pitfalls and explain the importance of the simple rules.

2 THE FIRST MEETING

Some key points:
- **Emphasize shared learning.**
- **Start by talking about the process.**
- **Give it a go.**

You have found your local expert. They can get you and your team started on an individual team basis, or you may be part of a workshop, with a number of teams present. The workshop approach has a number of attractions for organisations like Acute Trusts or Primary Care Trusts, since a number of teams can begin at the same time, and the idea of learning between teams can be encouraged. The shared learning within and between organisations is critical for the success of developing a culture of openness and reflection.

The format of the session is similar for individual teams and workshops, starting with a talk about the process, followed by 'giving it a go' in a safe facilitated environment. This inevitably has a powerful effect on the team members, who become committed to continuing the effort when they return to their working environment.

3   FACILITATION

It is debatable whether or not external facilitation is necessary to get started. The reality is probably that it depends on the team and the existing leadership skills. Some health care professionals are extremely adept at leadership and small group skills. Others are in need of going on a course! Clinical governance leads should be able to put teams in touch with facilitators. In large organisations there is sense in using one or two facilitators since it ensures consistency in the process of SEA.

4   SEVEN STEPS OF SIGNIFICANT EVENT AUDIT

1. Logging events
2. Creating the agenda
3. Managing the meeting
4. Discussing the event
5. Deciding the possible outcome
6. Writing up the meeting and reviewing the outcomes
7. Sharing the learning with others.

4.1   Logging events

It is best to log an event soon after it happens, when it is fresh in your mind. It is important to log episodes that went remarkably well and not just those not so good events. There is no one method for teams to log events. It is best that they chose a way that fits their style of work. Some teams use a book at the reception desk or nursing station, while others log them on the computer. What does not work is a general question about events in the last month: you only remember the catastrophes and exclude the important opportunities to celebrate successes.

Include any event that is anything other than routine for your team, especially where there is room for improvement or an opportunity for learning. These can be clinical and administrative. It is best that major adverse events, particularly relating to poor performance, are addressed through other existing channels. Events which occur in other organisations and have a bearing on you or your patients should be logged, since there may be potential learning for you as well as the originating organisation. For these events, try to invite someone with appropriate knowledge of the event from the other organisation to your team meeting.

Examples of clinical events could include:

- deaths in the last month,
- complications from a chronic disease,
- a case of meningitis or a teenage pregnancy.

Administrative examples could include:

- a problem with appointments,
- a complaint,
- computer coding problems,
- a dispensing error.

There is a temptation to discuss general issues, rather than specific named examples; complaints about access, rather than Mrs X's wheelchair getting stuck in the surgery door. However, because of the emotional connection, the specific case always leads to a better discussion and change is more likely.

There is increasing interest in the use of triggers for adverse incident reporting and learning. The triggers in general practice would identify a set of circumstances where there should be a team discussion. Examples of triggers could be:

- People under sixty who die from coronary heart disease
- Errors in warfarin control (INRs of over 5)
- Hospitalisations for people with asthma.

These cases need to be reviewed by the team to decide if any improvements could have been made. More work is required to identify the core set of triggers for various health care settings.

4.2   Creating the agenda

- Three days before the meeting, the person who has been chosen to chair the SEA meeting needs to collect all the events to produce the agenda, with sufficient time for team members to gather information about the events.
- Within the first couple of meetings, everyone should have the opportunity to present an event. If they are not included in the early stages, they may drift off and be difficult to re-engage.
- It is logical to have the important issues high on the agenda, and anything not addressed can be carried over to the next meeting. The first (and most important item) is 'Matters arising' from the last meeting.
- Often discussion about an event leads to further work away from the meeting by two or three people. This is the opportunity for them to feed back on their work, such as updating guidelines, and this has the effect of gaining ownership from the wider group.
- Even more importantly it ensures that people do what they say they will do, leading to genuine improvement in systems.
- It is unlikely that the team will discuss more than ten issues, and usually much less. As a general rule an event, which leads to discussion of more than ten minutes, requires further work at another time.

4.3   Managing the meeting

When encouraging teams to participate in Significant Event Audit, it is important to stress that the meeting is a substitute for an existing inter-professional meeting, not an addition.

Most teams welcome the opportunity of re-invigorating a team meeting which has lost its momentum. The meeting should last no more than an hour, preferably preceded by a sandwich, which emphasises the important social and supportive nature of the group.

For most teams, a meeting somewhere between monthly and two monthly seems about right. It is hard to identify the time (and sometimes the events) if meetings occur more frequently than monthly. If less frequent than two monthly, the group skills can be lost and it is like starting afresh each time.

For the more sceptical team members, you can convince them that this 'golden hour' of protected time will be extremely beneficial. Divert the phone and give yourself a break from continuous patient contact.

The chairperson of the meeting does not have to be the most senior team member. The team usually knows who has the best chairing skills. Often nurses make better chairpersons than doctors, probably because the meeting becomes less hierarchical. After all, flattening hierarchies is one of the aims of this type of team building. What is important is that the chairperson is able to balance the involvement of all group members as well as ensuring that discussion leads to action.

Organisations may need to think of running courses on small group and leadership courses, since for some, particularly clerical staff, group work is likely to be new to them.

Anyone who is part of the team delivering patient care should be invited to the SEA meeting. This should involve receptionists, nurses, physiotherapists and doctors, as well as any other people involved in individual cases. A key member of the team in an Accident & Emergency department was the porter. She often knew the best solution to a problem, but nobody had ever asked her before. In large teams, there is a temptation to invite representatives of professional groups. It is probably better to be inclusive, at the risk of having a large group. If someone is not in the team discussion, they will have difficulty owning the solutions. On a more positive note, the converse is definitely true, namely that if you are part of developing a solution to an adverse event, you will do things differently in the future.

For less confident team members, particularly if lower down in an organisation's hierarchy, strength in numbers may be important to give individuals confidence to speak out and develop ideas. More confident team members need to learn to value others' contributions. Their views are just as valid and probably more original.

Experts in group theory will tell you that group size is important, with a maximum of twelve for effective group functioning. In SEA, when people are already used to working in a team, the groups function well with larger numbers. Health care teams are often large, and efforts to split teams usually fail, since group members are inquisitive about the discussions in the other group, and it is hard to get ownership of someone else's solutions.

4.4   Discussing the event

The person most involved in an event should present the details, taking no longer than a couple of minutes. Some people, particularly in less powerful positions or new to the team, find this presentation difficult, especially if the event had less than ideal outcomes. There should be an opportunity for factual questions before a general discussion begins.

Some key points to bear in mind:
- **In the best tradition of team building, positive observations should precede more negative ones (Pendleton's rules).**
- **In even the direst of events, seek out something positive, which can always (or nearly always) be found.**
- **When coming up with solutions including systems changes, the ideas from the group are always gems, which must not be lost.**

> My partner in general practice is a hopeless timekeeper and always finishes his surgeries up to an hour late. Over the last 20 years, he has come up with at least 15 different models to make his surgery run to time. He has been known to run workshops on time management! None of his models worked. At an SEA meeting, following criticism from a disgruntled patient, the receptionist knew the answer and there have been no problems since.

Most issues can be resolved, with active chairmanship, within 10 minutes. As a rule of thumb, if the discussion is taking longer, it should be steered to another meeting at another time. It is important to use the 'golden hour' optimally. These meetings are taking up valuable time for busy people, who will disengage if they feel it is not worthwhile.

Early in the development of a Significant Event Audit team meeting, it is helpful if a senior team member (preferably a doctor) to be open and admit that a particular event could have been handled better. This gives the message to the rest of the team that it is OK to make a mistake as long as you learn from it. It is very hard for a ward clerk to start the process, since they would be worried about their prospects of long term employment. This important change of emphasis is at the heart of developing a 'no blame culture'.

Building on experience of investigating incidents, and extensively researched by Charles Vincent, a leading expert in investigating incidents in secondary care, the key issues to address are:

- **What happened?**
- **Where did it happen?**
- **When did it happen?**
- **How did it happen?**
- **Why did it happen?**
- **What action was taken or proposed?**
- **What impact did the event have?**
- **What factors did, or could have, minimised the impact of the event?**

Some or all of these questions may be relevant in discussing an event, and may form the basis of a minimum data set for the reporting of more serious adverse events. However the vast majority of agenda items discussed at a team SEA meeting are of the mild to moderate variety. These provide huge opportunities for learning, and yet are not of sufficient seriousness to be reported outside a team or organisation.

4.5 Deciding the possible outcomes

- Congratulations
- Immediate action
- Further work is called for
- No action

As a result of his ground-breaking research, Pringle came up with four outcomes of Significant Event Audit. Chapters 8 to 11 present short case studies of each of the outcomes in real-life settings, and here we will give a brief overview of each of the four.

4.5.1 Congratulations

The first and possibly the most important outcome is congratulations of success. There is no history of praising people or teams about good aspects of care. However, teams and individuals are frequently providing excellent care in difficult circumstances. Managing a bed crisis or a major disaster are all in a day's work for hard pressed professionals. Recognition of success in a team setting is a powerful team builder.

> At 10 am, a sensible mum asked to speak to a young general practitioner about her 4 year old child, who had a fever in the night. She contacted the out of hours service and was given routine advice. The mother said that her child was very drowsy and not at all well. The GP remembered that mum had declined the MMR, and just felt that she should see the child immediately rather than at the end of surgery. She visited and made a probable diagnosis of meningitis, got the husband to dial 999 and gave an ampoule of Penicillin. The child went straight to ITU due to shock, but made a full recovery. The paediatrician rang later in the day to say that but for her prompt action, the child would have died. The family gave the GP a bouquet of flowers. At the next SEA meeting, the case was discussed, and it was clear that the receptionist helped considerably to flag up the problem for the GP, not to mention with dealing with the rest of her surgery. Also the dispenser was responsible for having a system to check that the Penicillin in the GP's bag was in date.

There is frequently as much learning to be shared within the team from good events as not so good ones. The bonus is that the individual feels valued and, on a personal professional basis, knows they are doing their job well.

4.5.2   Immediate action

Highlighting an incident at a Significant Event Audit meeting may show that something has to be put right or improved straight away. The team sees the need, comes up with ideas, agrees the solution and agrees to act, leading to immediate change. Here may be a person nominated to implement the change. The team members own the change process which is a good predictor of the change becoming a permanent feature of the organisation. People unable to attend due to other commitments, shift work or holidays, need to be informed through a reporting process, but they will always be less committed to the particular change issue.

> Numerous patients in an Accident & Emergency department commented to a radiographer about the discomfort experienced while lying on trolleys, awaiting an X-ray. She raised the issue at a Significant Event Audit meeting, where the total absence of pillows on trolleys was discussed. The department manager agreed immediately that this should be rectified and now all trolleys have pillows.

Significant Event Audit is very effective at solving apparently little niggles, which no one had known how to address. These issues are usually only known to people who previously were unaware of mechanisms to flag up problems.

> A Health Authority had two large meeting rooms, one of which was in a separate building and required a secretary to guide visitors through complex corridors. A certain secretary was spending most of her time acting as a guide. This was brought to an SEA meeting, and now only internal meetings are held in the distant meeting room.

The effect to an organisation of people feeling that these little irritants can be solved is very liberating. You don't always have to do what you always did. Things can be improved – it is possible. The secretary who was spending her time as a guide is now much more productive in the office, but also very good at suggesting items for the agenda of SEA meetings!

4.5.3   Further work is called for – a potential topic for Quality Improvement

The third category as described by Pringle in 1995, include issues requiring further work, which would be amenable to **Clinical Audit**. In view of the broadening quality agenda, it was thought that an outcome purely leading to audit was limiting, and we should take advantage of other improvement techniques, like guideline production or adaptation, a care pathway or a PDSA cycle (Plan/Do/Study/Act). Discussion at an SEA meeting has identified an important issue which requires further work, probably by two or three people, away from the SEA team discussion. The discussion has probably taken ten minutes, and the meeting is in danger of being dominated by this one issue. At this stage the chairman should identify a small group of volunteers to further analyse and develop solutions that can be brought back to the next meeting.

> A fifty year-old patient with epilepsy died from an aspiration pneumonia following a grand mal seizure. The case was discussed at a general practice SEA meeting, resulting in one of the doctors and the practice nurse agreeing to do a revue of all people with epilepsy and updating the practice guidelines. They would report back to the next SEA meeting.

Bringing the issue back to the next meeting not only ensures that the task is done, but also allows feedback and subsequent ownership from the whole group. This gets round the usual problem of guidelines only being useful to the people who wrote them!

> A district nurse described her frustration at visiting an elderly patient who was discharged from the District General Hospital (DGH) on Friday evening. The good news was that they had informed her (this is not always the case). The bad news was that the medication sent out with the patient was only sufficient to last till Sunday. The outcome of the discussion was that the chairman would write to the Medical Director of the DGH to ensure that their discharge policy was reviewed to guarantee a minimum of three days medication is sent out with the patient.

This example demonstrates that the team is very dependent on other organisations. Solutions frequently lie outside the team, but that should not deter finding answers. A representative of the DGH could have been invited for this agenda item. Even more powerfully, why not invite the patient or carer?

Many problems in the NHS lie between organisations. SEA can be effective at addressing the gaps. The days of market forces and competition are fortunately behind us. Relationships between organisations are the key to improving the whole patient experience or 'patient journey'. Looking at significant events arising between organisations and learning from them can be a powerful stimulus to improve quality. Sadly, not all parties are similarly committed, or working at the same speed. This takes time.

4.5.4 No action

Not all significant events are amenable to change; there are times when experiences can be usefully expressed, but no action needs to be taken.

Sometimes these occasions can be especially important, representing as they do examples of team members' frustration – "Life's like that"… Providing a safe environment for listening and sharing has been shown to be a much-valued benefit of SEA.

So SEA enhances the quality of care directly by providing a forum for learning from the team's experiences, through its constituent individual members. Risk management can be addressed through immediate action, improvements initiated, enquiries set up, and relevant topics for improvement projects identified.

At the same time, SEA provides an opportunity to team build, or to strengthen existing teams. Working together on quality improvement generates mutual understanding and an atmosphere of trust, which can itself begin to create a setting in which delicate areas such as the exploration of deficiencies in performance can take place. All of which adds up to good reasons to try it!

4.6   Writing up the meeting and reviewing the outcomes

The mere fact that a report of a Significant Event Audit meeting is written up and circulated amongst those who attended and those who were unable to attend, makes an important statement about the importance of SEA. The process belongs to the whole team and the wide dissemination of a report is a means of reinforcing the change process. Most teams use a standardised form (see Figure 2). The most frequently forgotten aspect is a review date. Are we doing what we said we should do?

The report can also be used as evidence of learning in individuals' personal learning portfolios. Also an individual leaning need may have been identified, and the review process can be used to ensure that this need has been met. The individual may need help to find a suitable course, which may have resource implications for the team.

If patients make a criticism of the service and are made aware that the SEA meeting will be used to discuss an improvement, the report (or just the appropriate section) can be used as evidence of change. Patients like to be involved with service improvement.

"All I wanted was to make sure that it would not happen to someone else".

Significant Event Audit

Meeting date _____

Present _____

_____

_____

_____

_____

_____

_____

Topic	Action to be taken	Key individual(s)	Date implemented	Review date

Figure 2. Suggested regular Team SEA recording form

Some participants have been concerned about the legal status of the SEA minutes. Like any other medical documentation, they may be required in some circumstances for legal purposes. Rather than counting against an individual or team, they are more likely to act in favour of the team for taking a proactive learning approach to a particular adverse event. The minutes only complement information available elsewhere in medical and nursing records.

4.7   Sharing the learning with others

For every catastrophe, there are over three hundred near misses, giving opportunities for the team to learn and develop improved systems. This reservoir of opportunities could be vastly increased if teams learnt from other teams' near misses. If there is no strong history in the NHS of learning from our own mistakes in a blame-free environment, there is certainly no history of learning from other people's mistakes. In *An Organisation with a Memory* the author suggests a national database of incidents, as exists in the airline industry. However the database will only be effective if the culture becomes more open, in order to encourage openness.

Within some Primary Care Trusts, reports of SEA meetings are regularly passed to the clinical governance lead in a confidential environment. This requires a strong trusting relationship between teams and the clinical governance lead, which takes time to develop. The airline industry experience is that anonymity increases willingness to report incidents. Early pilot projects of sharing learning about adverse incidents in primary care organisations indicate that patient anonymity is far more important than practice anonymity. It is essential that general practice or team details are treated confidentially by the Clinical Governance lead.

These pilots have also demonstrated that PCT-wide meetings, for example of practice clinical governance leads, are an opportunity for sharing the learning from incidents in a powerful way. With suitable safeguards, these lessons could be shared in a clinical governance or PCT newsletter. However hearing about an incident from someone involved will always have more impact than a newsletter or guideline. Similarly, locally developed systems of sharing learning will be more effective than national solutions. Figure 3 shows a suggested format for flagging issues

Significant Event Audit reporting framework

Meeting date _____

Team* _____

_____

_____

_____

_____

_____

_____

Topic

_____

_____

_____

_____

Action to be taken

_____

_____

_____

_____

Implementation date _____

Share learning with other teams?   Yes/No

*Inserting team name is optional

Figure 3. Suggested form to flag potential shared learning

for shared learning, which can be easily modified from Figure 2, by deleting a couple of columns.

There are many barriers to the sharing of learning from incidents, which added together give the impression of being overwhelming. If you are feeling brave, make the suggestion to a group of senior professionals, and they will come up with the difficulties. Experience suggests that you have to give it a go with a small number of willing teams (the early adopters) and then demonstrate that it can be safe and beneficial to patients and professionals alike.

There is a conflict about what incident should be reported (or shared). The national database, as outlined in *An Organisation with a Memory* will be concentrating on more major incidents, whereas some of the greater benefits in terms of sharing learning may be about more mundane issues e.g. aspects of Health & Safety, including needle-stick injuries or chemical spillages. SEA in many ways is more effective with the more minor incidents (or near misses), rather than major ones, particularly where there are legal or poor performance issues to contend with. In an organisation where all teams use SEA as a tool for improving quality, there is an opportunity to learn not just within a team, but also between teams and between organisations.

It is important to remember that the learning from adverse events at team and organisation level is far more worthwhile than smart national reporting structures. Politicians can only put structures in place – teams can learn and improve their patients' experience.

Chapter 3

The history and development of Significant Event Audit

1 WHERE DID SIGNIFICANT EVENT AUDIT COME FROM?

The most recognisable forebear of SEA is the critical incident technique as developed by Colonel John C. Flanagan, chief of the Psychological Branch, Research Division, Office of the Air Surgeon, part of the United States Air Force. A programme was set up in the summer of 1941 to develop procedures for the selection and classification of bomber air crews. Prior to this programme, there was a high drop-out rate after the initial training of pilots and crew. They collected information about the circumstances of successful and unsuccessful bombing raids, to learn about the characteristics of specific roles and particularly about leadership. The focus was on people, getting the right skills into the team.

It is interesting to reflect that SEA has been seen as a tool for learning about events, both good and bad. Increasingly it is also a vehicle for looking after team members, valuing and understanding their contribution, and identifying individual development needs. The development of SEA is mirroring the critical incident technique.

Towards the end of 1944, when large numbers of air crew were returning home, there was a large scale project run by Wickert and Flanagan, gathering specific information of effective and ineffective behaviour in respect of accomplishing assigned missions. From this they developed the 'critical requirements' of combat leadership.

The top five categories were:

1. Consideration of men's welfare. Went to "bat" for men's safety, comfort, food etc.

2. Ability to mix with subordinates. Had a knack of being one of the boys.
3. Unusual proficiency in his rated speciality and knowledge of his equipment. Knew his planes.
4. Sharing of dangers. Flew large percentage of raids.
5. Approachability. Easy to approach with new ideas.

Most, but not all these skills, are applicable in SEA!

After the war, the initiative of critical incident technique was continued in the University of Pittsburgh and the American Institute of Research. It was used by the General Motors Corporation in 1949, and this was the first example of collecting incidents on a day-to-day basis as a continuous record of job performance. The approach spread to civilian airlines and also Westinghouse, where they noted that emphasising good events increased the reporting of incidents greatly. This important message needs to be re-learnt today.

2   ORIGINS IN HEALTH CARE

The first example of the critical incident technique in health care was in the Pittsburgh School of Dentistry at about the same time.

In health care, there has been a long history of learning from experience. In his seminal paper 'The Critical Incident Technique', Flanagan paid tribute to the work of Sir Francis Galton in the 1880s. Although more famous as the father of eugenics and being Charles Darwin's cousin, as a medical student he observed the differing outcomes of an array of surgeons in accident departments in London. Sadly he did not continue this work when he inherited a large legacy and did not qualify as a doctor!

There has been a long tradition in hospitals of learning from adverse incidents in morbidity and mortality meetings, and more recently through confidential enquiries e.g. the Confidential Enquiry into Perioperative Deaths (CEPOD). In general practice, the more informal approach of discussing cases over coffee or in corridors, is well established. By the 1980s, a few GPs were beginning to use SEA in a more formal way, linked to vocational training. Professor Mike Pringle moved SEA centre-stage with the publication by the Royal College of General Practice of his Occasional Paper on Significant Event Auditing in 1995.

As well as describing the process of SEA, he also compared the effectiveness of SEA and conventional audit.

3   CONFUSING TERMINOLOGY – WHAT SEA IS NOT

Significant Event Audit has a specific meaning, which describes ongoing inter-professional team learning activity from events both good and not so good. It is not the right place for serious incidents or issues of poor performance which are better addressed through other channels. The commonest misunderstanding is that SEA is a one off meeting to discuss an adverse event. In mental health services, this is generally known as a Critical Incident Review. It is quite correct that such a meeting should be held soon after a serious adverse incident, which may serve a number of purposes, including learning from the event, supporting team members and possibly discussing possible legal and procedural consequences.

A *Critical Incident Case Study* is a term used by nurses who are involved in an adverse incident and use it as a topic for reflection. This would be included in their personal learning portfolio, or discussed during their clinical supervision.

Both of the above uses of the words *Critical Incident* are important but they mean something different to Significant Event Audit.

4   WHAT NOT TO BRING TO SEA MEETINGS

It takes at least four meetings to develop a level of trust in the group that can cope with issues that are moderately adverse. They need to be well balanced with good events. When first discussing something which could have been managed better, it is easier that the case involves someone senior. They can more easily demonstrate that is OK to be open about an adverse incident than someone more junior. In primary care, it is better for a GP to present such a case. A receptionist would be more focused on keeping her job! Incidents which involve aspects of poor performance are best dealt with through other existing channels. If, during the course of a team meeting, poor performance issues become apparent, these concerns should be dealt with away from the meeting. It is not easy to be consistent in the message that it is good to be open about incidents and there really is a 'no-blame' culture.

5   SUITABLE SETTINGS FOR SIGNIFICANT EVENT AUDIT

Due to the dissemination of the findings of Pringle's work through a series of regional workshops, the initial wave of enthusiasm in Significant Event Audit has been in primary care. With the development of clinical governance, a number of leaders with an interest in improving patient care have seen the potential for SEA. Many Primary Care Groups and Trusts have worked with all their practices to ensure that regular SEA meetings are taking place. It has been the vehicle for bringing together a number of small practices to share the learning from adverse events. The development of clinical governance in primary care has been linked to the spread of SEA. It was seen as achievable and beneficial in a number of ways for a range of health care professionals, probably because it was recognised as a way of addressing everyday issues in a straightforward way.

Departments in **secondary care** have used the technique with great effect, although there are some interesting issues about the introduction of the process. (See chapter 10 for more details.)

6   SOME KEY LESSONS

Some of the lessons that have been learnt are:

6.1   Leadership

Although the initial urge seems to be for consultants to drive this process, this is not always the best strategy. In an Accident & Emergency Department, the enthusiastic, dynamic consultant got the meetings off the ground. The meetings were well attended by doctors, but not particularly by nurses. They were seen to be useful, but not meeting the needs of the whole department. The leadership switched to the nurse manager and suddenly the nurse attendance improved dramatically. All the doctors still came, but the meetings were more effective.

With well established groups, rotation of the role of chair may have advantages. It certainly needs to be discussed by the team. The same goes for the person with the secretarial duties.

6.2   Timing

In most hospital departments and wards, you can't close the frontdoors for an hour of training. This is invariably the first barrier which hospital teams perceive. Now that it appears to be accepted that you can't expect front-line workers to deliver care and improve services at the same time, hospital leaders have to come up with ways of creating protected time for hard-pressed professionals. Some of the solutions have included meeting at the change-over of shifts. It is probably unrealistic to aim for one hundred percent attendance. It is more important to get a core group of people with a good understanding of the concept of SEA. The timing of meetings should be made around accommodating nursing needs, since they are the major part of the workforce, with least flexibility.

Most professional groups and departments have set times of learning. When introducing SEA, it is important to sell the learning potential and the meetings themselves are part of learning. Copies of the minutes should be kept in the individual team member's learning portfolio.

6.3   Incentives

Sandwiches at the beginning of a meeting, provided by the organisation, are always well received. The gesture suggests that senior management value their staff and want to support the development of a reflective culture. This will be a challenge for Trust boards, who for a number of years have been guided down a line of savings, and the result has been that it is hard, particularly for nurses, to feel that they are valued when they have to pay for parking, uniform and food. Significant Event Audit is an important tool to enable teams to build mutual respect, and organisations to respect their teams.

6.4   Reports

The documentation of SEA meetings poses a fundamental paradox which needs to be discussed in each team and directorate. How do you create an open 'no-blame' culture and have a reporting mechanism to your departmental clinical governance lead, and through them to the chief executive? This is a complex issue, which depends on trust built up over a number of years. It is relatively easy to ensure patient confidentiality when the report goes out of the team setting, but not so simple, or necessarily desirable, to ensure confidentiality for health care staff.

When introducing SEA, it is wise to sell it as a team activity, which is owned by all. It is everyone's chance to raise issues, which will probably lead to real change. This is where the culture change takes place. The reporting mechanism is a secondary issue which, if handled sensitively, is an added bonus.

Internal circulation of the report of the meeting is particularly important for those unable to attend the meeting, e.g. night staff and those who can't be spared from front-line duties. It is hard for these people to feel part of solutions which were generated during the SEA meeting. The chairman of the meeting may need to talk through some of the outcomes, particularly if there are consequences for the individual.

There has been experience of SEA in **prison health care units**. In an environment of isolation from the rest of health care, there are some particular issues about the introductory process. The level of team-working in the NHS is not mirrored in prison health care and so there is probably a need for external facilitation. Shift working is also an obstacle, but there is dedicated time for learning. The support of the prison governor is just as important of the support of a chief executive in a Trust. There is sometimes a pervading feeling that it is not possible to change anything – a difficult climate for SEA to thrive.

SEA has also been used by **social service departments**. Their front desk staff are frequently faced with difficult clients, and SEA has been used to discuss issues of personal security, diffusing stressful situations and improving ways of calling for help. Social care staff are frequently to be found participating in health care team meetings, so are well used to developing team solutions. This is particularly true in the fields of mental health, and dealing with older people.

7   THE EMERGING MODEL

Significant Event Audit is not new, and has been developed and improved over time. The introduction of clinical governance into the NHS has given SEA a legitimacy, as a key foundation stone of quality. If you are the chief executive, you value it as a risk management tool. If you are a team leader, you are attracted by the learning potential of the meetings, and if you are a team member, the support from other professionals is what keeps you attending.

The recent developments in SEA have been in defining the links with Quality Improvement. SEA identifies the issues which need to be improved. Quality Improvement brings the systems thinking that enables the move away from individual blame. A focus on improving systems leads to improved outcomes. In general, errors tend to occur due to imperfect systems rather than imperfect people. It is OK to be involved in and discuss an adverse event, as long as lessons are learnt and systems improved.

The potential of SEA as the bedrock of a pyramid for adverse incident reporting is also being discussed, as organisations are introducing SEA into all teams. There may well be added value from including patients in particular agenda items, if the team feels that this appropriate. An alternative model may be to include some patient representatives (or 'critical friends') at all meetings so as to encourage them to work with professional staff, and add their ideas to develop smarter solutions. This is an area to be further researched.

SEA helps to develop an open reflective culture, which concentrates on improving systems rather than individual blame. This is achieved by addressing everyday issues to which everyone can relate. Wise leaders of health and social care organisations will make the time for such an important activity.

Chapter 4

Significant Event Audit, learning and improving

1   PERSONAL LEARNING PLANS

All healthcare professionals in the NHS will require personal learning plans and will need to keep a portfolio with evidence of learning. This is usually in paper format but will increasingly be electronic. The underlying principles of the personal learning plan is the Learning Cycle developed by Kolb in the 1960s, and refined and adapted for health care professionals further, since then (see Figure 4).

When identifying learning needs, the commonest response is that it is difficult to identify what you don't know. Significant Event Audit can be of great help. Since SEA is based in everyday practice, dealing with real

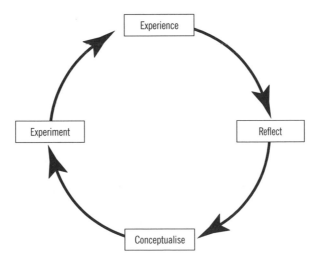

Figure 4. The learning cycle

issues, it is very good at identifying learning needs. The learning cycle begins with **Experience**, followed by the **Reflection** phase. Both of these elements are part of the SEA meeting, with the added advantage that both phases may be team activities as well as personal learning.

The emphasis of learning in the past has been on the individual, but with the recognition that most patient care is delivered by teams, there is a shift of emphasis on team learning. This has a number of benefits. Firstly, there will be consistency in the standard of care given, and secondly, the team is able to discuss who should develop particular skills. In a general practice, the team can move away from 'all knowing everything' – an increasingly impossible task. One practice nurse and general practitioner can take responsibility to know the latest evidence on diabetes care, while others concentrate on other chronic diseases. **Conceptualising** new solutions for old problems is at the heart of learning and innovating. The latter is an increasingly important skill, when the relentless increase in pressure on the health service makes it imperative that delivery of care needs to be different – you can't just keep working harder and harder. The final part of the cycle is **Experiment**. This may seem a step too far for a number of teams! However, it fits exactly with what is required to modernise services in the NHS. It is OK to do things differently. It is also OK for some experiments to fail, as long as lessons are learnt.

There is an uncanny similarity between the learning cycle and the PDSA cycle, developed by Nolan and Langley in the late 1980s. Again, SEA identifies the issues for improvement/learning. After discussion at the SEA meeting, an individual or a small group will be identified to look at a particular issue, and if necessary begin to develop a change to an existing system. This may be an improved method of infection control, based on latest evidence.

The neat aspect of the PDSA cycle is that it is very empowering. Rather than enter into a mind-numbing clinical audit of the next two hundred patients to prove that there really is a problem, the PDSA cycle encourages a change to systems once a problem is identified. It also encourages little changes often, with a series of cycles over a short time frame. Nolan has very cleverly devised three very important fundamental questions.

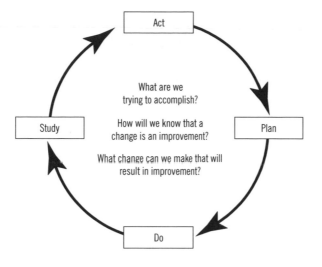

Figure 5. The model for improvement

1.1 What are we trying to accomplish?

This is the Aim of the project. If you don't have a tight aim, you won't improve anything. This is probably the most important stage of the whole process and deserves more emphasis than in the past. This is true whatever the setting. You don't stop smoking or lose weight unless you set a specific aim, such as 'I'll stop smoking on No Smoking Day', or 'I'll lose 5 kilograms before the holiday in St Tropez (or Bognor Regis!)'.

1.2 How will we know that a change is an improvement?

This is the Measurement aspect of the project, enabling you to tell whether things are getting better. Is the level of hospital acquired infections improving, and is the monthly rate of methicillin-sensitive staphyloccus aureus the right measure?

1.3 What changes can we make that will result in an improvement?

Ideas to solve problems are like precious gems. Solutions were traditionally generated by senior managers, and they were rarely successful. The people who usually know the answers are the front-line staff, but they were rarely asked. SEA involves all the team, so is an excellent place to capture ideas, which lead to successful solutions. The reception staff can tell you the number of appointment slots you need to provide on any day of the week, but traditional thinking dictates that the doctors set the number of consultations and clinics.

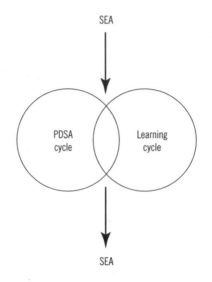

Figure 6. Improvement and learning cycles

Thinking about learning and improvement cycles at the same time emphasises the intricate links between Continuous Quality Improvement and Continuous Professional Development. The processes are so similar. They are both closely aligned to Significant Event Audit, which anchors both processes in the daily life of health care workers. The topics are identified in SEA meetings and progress reports are brought back to the meeting. This has the twin functions of keeping the team up-to-date, and also checking that identified work is completed – change really can happen!

Continuous Quality Improvement encourages small changes to be made, with frequent measurements. The completion of a number of improvement (**PDSA**) cycles is a change from the more laboured and often incomplete clinical audit cycles. The beginning of the improvement cycle relies heavily on ideas from the team (**PLAN**), which are then incorporated into an improved system, which is tested (**DO**). This may well

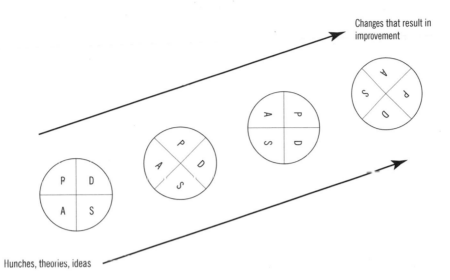

Changes that result in improvement

Hunches, theories, ideas

Figure 7. PDSA cycles after T. Nolan et al.

lead to an improvement (**STUDY**), which can be further improved by incorporating more ideas (**ACT**). Some ideas may not lead to improvement, and these will be discarded. There is as much to be learnt from ideas that don't lead to change as in those that do (probably more)!

Chapter 5

Sustaining Significant Event Audit

1   WHY IS IT IMPORTANT?

After all the effort of getting SEA started in the team, with or without external facilitation, it is common to experience a honeymoon period for three or four months. At about six months, the SEA meeting seems to have lost momentum. It is surprisingly common to hear these stories, and a number of follow-up workshops have been held to address the issues and think of strategies that teams may find useful.

2   COMMON PROBLEMS

2.1   Leadership and chairing meetings

It may be best to have two people sharing the leadership, so that if an event is discussed involving one the other can chair. The facilitator/chair may need help – training and formal support should be available. Similarly communication skills training should also be offered.

Rotation of the chairmanship should be discussed by the team. If a natural SEA leader has been identified, the group may vote for the status quo. The development of these skills should be nurtured in more than one individual. Think of succession planning.

2.2   Ground rules

These should be the basic rules that all team members sign up to.

- SEA is constructive, with a 'no-blame' approach giving mutual support to team members.
- The meetings are confidential, and only patient anonymous reports leave the team.
- The meeting should have an agenda, with some space for the inclusion of 'hot topics'.
- Agreed actions are progressed or completed before the next meeting.
- Never discuss an event without all key individuals present.
- The individual involved in an incident comments first and then others may join in the discussion.
- Always look for some element of an event to celebrate.
- The agenda has balance of good and not so good events.
- There is a report written after all meetings and circulated to all team members.

2.3   Size of group

It is difficult to get the balance right between including everyone and not making the meeting too big (which makes it uncomfortable for some people to speak out). It may depend on the issues being discussed. Perhaps each team should ask what it is trying to achieve? What is the right team to achieve the purpose? Has the team got the right group and the group right?

Conventional group theory dictates an optimal size of 8–12. Experience with SEA shows that larger groups can work, probably because the individuals work with one another anyway. Attempts to run smaller groups in parallel have usually failed, because people like to be involved in all the issues, and anyway, would you own the other group's solutions?

2.4   Actions too great a task

Action points can include future intentions and ideas – you don't have to sort everything out in one go! If people outside the team are involved, the team should feel able to invite them to join in. Projects identified by SEA should be undertaken by two or three people. If an individual is nominated for a task, there is often reluctance to put significant events on the agenda. Beware the feeling that SEA always generates extra work for people. These small project teams may need managerial or audit support. It is OK to carry forward action points, as long as progress is being made. However, it is important to review action points on a regular, perhaps half yearly, basis.

2.5 Overcoming fear

All members of the team, however senior or junior should have an opportunity of attending (or be represented at) an SEA meeting. However, a number of junior staff are not used to team meetings or being listened to. They should be given support or the chance to practise presenting an event prior to the meeting. Smaller groups will be less threatening. Also a healthy balance of congratulation and improvement outcomes is sure to help.

Like relationships, SEA meetings have to be worked at. Every so often, they get into trouble and may need external help. There should be assistance for leadership development facilitation, small group skills and communication available to all teams.

Chapter 6

Significant Event Audit and adverse incident reporting

1 BACKGROUND

As a result of a series of recurrent serious adverse incidents, there have been a number of national initiatives to develop a reporting mechanism and share the subsequent learning from these incidents. Work in the United States and Australia has been particularly useful, as has experience from other fields, especially the civil airlines industry, enabling the Chief Medical Officer, Professor Liam Donaldson, to publish his widely acclaimed discussion document *An Organsiation with a Memory.* This has been followed by *Building a Safer NHS for Patients* in April 2001.

There is a world wide recognition that at times of high risk activity in health care, adverse events are inevitable. What is important is that these events should be recorded, analysed and learned from, not only by the originating organisation, but by the whole NHS. To encourage this willingness to report incidents, a more open sharing culture is necessary, and is only achievable if a systems approach to problems, rather than the old blame and train method, is universally adopted in the NHS.

There are three important issues to address:

■ getting the culture right;
■ developing a reporting system;
■ sharing the learning.

These can all be discussed at local as well as national levels.

2   GETTING THE CULTURE RIGHT

The publication of erudite documents does not change culture, nor in general do national initiatives. For health care workers to begin to report adverse events, what ever the size, it is important for them to appreciate that their approach has the full support of the whole of their organisation at all levels, and that a disciplinary approach will not follow, except in cases of poor performance. Once an organisation is able to demonstrate that it will really adopt a systems approach, then this news travels very fast through the organisation. You only need a few examples to begin to change culture. The ideal position to be in is when people phone the medical director to ask whether a particular event is sufficiently serious to be reported.

In many ways, it is much easier to change culture around less serious adverse events. There is less likely to be concerns of poor performance, so staff are more open, and more likely to offer ideas to improve the system. This is the territory of Significant Event Audit. The regular multi-professional meeting is the ideal place to develop these systems improvements, and the resultant culture change. For very serious adverse event, there are 300 near misses. For every serious event, there are miriads of mild and moderate events, with opportunities to improve and systems to develop. There is no lack of material! Wherever the health care setting, there are teams that can use SEA to develop an open reflective improving culture.

This process won't happen by itself and needs to be managed and facilitated. This costs money, but such an investment will show rapid dividends by reducing waste, not to mention the reduced litigation by having safer systems.

3   DEVELOPING A REPORTING SYSTEM

By sharing the experiences of other countries, it will be possible to set up a national reporting framework. Initially, it will be necessary to be clear about definitions, and what constitutes an event worthy of being reported. Inevitably, there will have to be a cut off-point, but it is imperative to stress that just because some issue is not considered serious enough to be entered in the national register does not mean that there is no learning. Again SEA is better placed to pick up the issues not reported

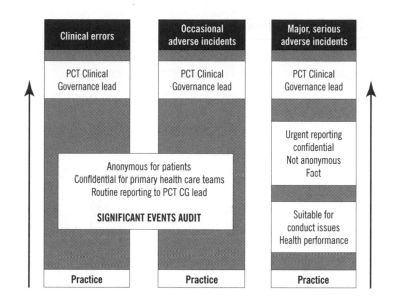

Figure 8. Logging adverse incidents and clinical errors

to the national register, because it will be less threatening, easier to involve the team, and more able to develop an open reflective culture.

It has yet to be decided how the reporting system will work, and how it will link to existing mechanisms. Health care organisations, both in primary and secondary care will have an obligation to report incidents. In general practice, the self-employed status of the doctor may be a political barrier to openeness at the beginning.

Once the event is logged on to a national data base, there will be a need to develop a standardised data collection tool, as well as an agreed approach to root cause analysis. The data base will be able to identify recurring themes both in this country and abroad. One of the first areas to be developed, since it accounts for at least a quarter of the adverse incidents, is drug error. Again, it is important to build on existing, well respected systems like the yellow card system of the Committee on Safety of Medicines (CSM).

4   SHARING THE LEARNING

Whether or not the event was sufficiently serious for reporting to the national register, there is a universal cycle of improvement.

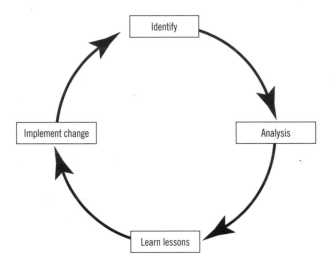

Figure 9. A cycle of improvement

Of course, this is the Significant Event Audit cycle, the improvement (PDSA) cycle and the Kolb Learning cycle. The learning from a local event, which goes to SEA meeting is likely to be instantaneous. The people involved in the incident will be part of the debate about improving systems. Locally generated ideas will be integral to the local solution. This will lead to real change, as well as reinforcement of a cultural change.

Learning shared within a health care organisation, either an Acute Trust or Primary Care Trust, can also be a powerful force for improvement. To witness the learning from someone involved in an adverse event is the next best thing to being integrally involved! There is beginning to be experienced in this type of shared learning between clinical governance leads in general practices within a PCT. It must be remembered that there have been many years of isolation for the majority of practices, with no history of openness between neighbouring practices, who, after all, were in competition.

For events reported through the national reporting mechanism, the learning will be rather more protracted. This is often appropriate when serious issues are concerned. Although there will be a local root cause analysis, solutions may depend on similar incidents in other places, and it will be harder for people in the originating organisation to own the learning. Paradoxically, those involved in an incident will always gain more from learning from an adverse event, and the organisation will be a safer place. The National Patient Safety Agency (NPSA), which is responsible for the reporting mechanism, will need to work hard at the disssemination and implementation process to ensure maximum learning from adverse events. However, the NPSA will always be more effective than local teams at being able to have influence with manufacturers of devices or software computer companies to make crucial changes.

Part 2

Chapter 7

Looking for the evidence: observing Significant Event Audit in practice

1 INTRODUCTION

In this chapter we intend to discuss the impact of SEA by presenting three of our research studies in which we explored the use of SEA in two different health care environments. We will start the chapter by placing the work in the context of what is known about SEA before presenting the details of each separate study. Finally, we will conclude by drawing out the main messages that these three pieces of work teach us about the experience of this process and technique within primary care and prison health care.

2 THE CONTEXT

The earlier chapters explore the historical development of SEA as a technique in industry and latterly in health care. In these chapters, we have highlighted the seminal research that shaped the process and technique. In terms of the application of SEA in modern health care, we have indicated that Pringle and his colleagues drew the threads together in their study of the feasibility and potential of SEA in primary care during the mid 1990s. They are credited for describing the method, surveyed its use and comparing it to conventional audit. Pringle et al concluded that the technique's strengths could be summarised as:

■ its focus on outcomes,

- relevance to practice and practical problems,
- width of application; and
- team building qualities.

Amongst potential drawbacks the authors identified:

- possible superficiality;
- emotional demands on and threats to individuals; and
- training requirements and challenges to the team.

As we have indicated earlier, the importance, worth and relevance of SEA within health care was established by this work.

Despite promising beginnings, and for those developing SEA and extending its application in the conviction that the technique addresses a substantial part of the Clinical Governance agenda, crucial questions remain to be asked. Original research on the benefits as perceived by the participants themselves, is lacking. Whilst the technique of SEA has been well described and there is evidence of SEA producing follow-through into needs assessment and commissioning, the actual group processes and the individual experience remain poorly detailed. We would suggest that whilst there is some empirical evidence to support the particular model of SEA that has been advocated and widely adopted, few efforts have been made to evaluate:

- the benefits to the participants involved in SEA
- the extent to which it meets (or fails to meet) the needs of participants
- the personal and professional risks that SEA might hold for individuals
- possible strategies and techniques to facilitate the process of SEA
- the contribution of SEA to team building, individual professional development and quality assurance.

We will describe two studies of SEA in primary care and one in the prison health care system. The first, a preliminary investigation, produced guidance in identifying the barriers and enablers to facilitating the optimal implementation of SEA in primary care. The second enquiry follows up the preliminary study by observing the implementation and process of

SEA in a primary care practice. The final study explores the development of the process in the prison health care system. We will now move on to describe each of these in detail.

3   THE PRELIMINARY STUDY

In this preliminary study, we set about exploring the use of SEA within primary care teams. Specifically, we aimed to:

- describe and document individual team members' perceptions of SEA,
- on the basis of these perceptions, develop suggestions to improve the process.

3.1   Data collection

Data were collected through a series of 12 one-to-one interviews. Pools of potential participants were drawn from established SEA groups in three different primary care practices. Subjects were selected to provide a representative from each of the occupational groups within the primary care team and to represent the wider community team. Each interview was tape-recorded. The interview schedule was designed to elicit descriptive and explanatory information representing the interviewee's interpretation of the experience of SEA.

3.2   Participant profile

Study participants were divided into two main groups; practice-employed staff (two practice managers, two GPs, two practice nurses and two receptionists) and community staff who played an active role in practice life (one district nurse, one health visitor, one community psychiatric nurse and one community physiotherapist). The aim of this sampling procedure was to provide a voice to individuals within the practice and to those who sometimes were viewed as outsiders. Ages ranged from 37 to 58 years (mean 46 years), and eight subjects were female. Only three participants worked full-time, the remainder working between 12 and 30 hours per week. Their length of time in their post ranged from 2 to 18 years (mean 8.6 years).

3.3   Results and discussion

All of the interviews were analysed using Grounded Theory. Table 1 presents the distilled themes as described above. We now address each category in turn.

Table 1. Results of grounded theory analysis grouped under two core headings

Perceptions of SEA	Facilitating the process of SEA
1. Advantages of SEA	1. Rules + guidelines
2. Disadvantages of SEA	2. Commitment/ownership
3. Concerns	3. Selection of topics
4. Conflicts	4. Leadership
5. Motivation	5. Debriefing
6. Resolutions and solutions	6. Censoring and vetting
7. Management of the process	

3.3.1   Perceptions of SEA by participants

3.3.1.1 Advantages

Participants welcomed the opportunity, indeed permission, that SEA gave them to discuss problems and difficulties, as well as suggestions and advice. These individuals could relate such discussions to:

- team building;
- the creation of trust;
- mutual understanding; and
- appreciation of other members' contributions.

As a result, the work environment was enhanced and a better quality service could be offered, which itself further improved morale. Participants enjoyed the multidisciplinary format, offering opportunities to learn about others' experiences and opinions, to work together to problem solve and to resolve conflict, often without personalization. Members could see how SEA encouraged individual development both within and alongside the team.

"I think they [SEA meetings] could benefit the running of the practice, initiate improvements in quality and care of patients, and also perhaps improve relationships between staff, increase awareness of others' roles. I think they present a challenge, make people stop and think rather than just jogging along and also perhaps make people feel more part of the whole team, so everyone's got a chance to voice an opinion".

Practice Nurse

3.3.1.2 Disadvantages

■ Pringle and his colleagues suggested that SEA may have a number of potential drawbacks, including its superficial, threatening and emotionally demanding nature.

■ In addition, they proposed the view there may be difficulties in structuring the meetings, that some issues may be difficult to resolve and that there may be a need for extra training of staff. In the current study some members, particularly those employed by the doctors and apparently lower in the hierarchy, felt vulnerable in speaking out, especially if their contribution might be seen as critical of those perceived to be of higher status.

■ SEA represented a new and often uncomfortable experience for most of the team (in general, least so for the GPs), who found the critical process generally disconcerting and could be embarrassed by revelations of other members' shortcomings. There was a Pandora's box fear: that lifting the lid might release uncontainable pressures with unexpected consequences.

■ Finding the time for the meeting, especially when part-time staff had to make special arrangements to attend, posed practical difficulties. Even when this could be resolved, these members often found they had to carry straight on at work, or to go home, without adequate opportunity to talk things over.

"… It's quite a short period of time for some sensitive issues. Especially when we've all got surgery and things to do afterwards."

GP

3.3.1.3 Concerns

■ Members were uncertain about boundaries and anxious not to overstep margins. While the traditional demarcated roles within primary care might (and many would say ought to) be abandoned temporarily during the SEA meeting, it might be difficult to return to the *ancien regime* immediately afterwards – until next time.

■ Employed staff, in particular, worried about who was to lead SEA: without sufficiently strong and sympathetic chairing they felt vulnerable.

■ All staff feared the 'hornets' nest': it may be better to let some things be. Even when some difficult issues can be tackled, they may not be resolved adequately: "we still have to work together". As a result, SEA sometimes confined itself to safe areas, some of which appeared trivial and were dealt with in a superficial manner.

Non-doctors were concerned that GPs' topics might dominate the agenda.

> "… if we're going to start playing around with things that are quite emotional, then I think you've got to have somebody who's skilled within that group to recognise it. So… you've got to have somebody who's used to team work, knows how to start and end things and to intervene to keep everybody safe, because it's all very well us going round and doing these things, but if you're going to cause damage to the team because of it, then that's not going to solve any problems, it's just going to create more."
>
> Practice Nurse

3.3.1.4 Conflicts

Employed staff experienced a conflict in roles: they found it difficult to behave as equals during the meeting and then to return to 'employee status'. If the GP is your employer, it can be hard to speak out honestly. Other, externally employed, staff were differently stressed, with loyalties to the GPs and their own management structure sometimes in conflict. Some members (particularly nurses) felt their first loyalty was to their own staff group or discipline, which could interfere with SEA. In addition, there could be a conflict between personal and professional matters for various participants.

"I know that we've been told how the meetings should work, that everyone should be completely frank, and it's confidential and whatever happens in the room is only for that particular time, and I think that, in all honesty, most of us feel that if we were to be picky with somebody in there, it would actually be very difficult to actually come out and work with them… because of that, we have probably not been freely discussing the things that we should be."

Receptionist

3.3.1.5 Motivation

The selection of topics affected motivation. Because the leaders were more inclined to choose events that involved them, clinical GP topics could dominate SEA, particularly at first. This could alienate non-clinical staff.Certainly some members felt more motivated to contribute than others. GPs' motivation was increased by PGEA approval for attending (with no similar reward for other groups) and a social benefit. Others with less need for the social contacts felt less motivated. These might be receptionists, who were sometimes able to talk about their work problems as they worked, and so had less need for SEA.

Because the initiative for SEA often came from the GPs, their motivation to attend, contribute and make the meetings successful was often greater than that of other members, who occasionally saw the exercise as imposed. There was a danger of a vicious circle developing, with those attending dominating the proceedings and thus making SEA even less attractive for the non-attenders. It was particularly important for 'external' attached workers (community psychiatric nurses for example) to see relevant topics to motivate them to attend.

However, it was appreciated that the discussion of an event by those involved was a motivating experience and this encouraged people to attend the next time.

"The last couple I didn't bother [attending], because I was so busy and I didn't really, I haven't anything to give and yes, what was being said by other people didn't relate to me… I only do 18 hours and, [I'm] quite pushed, so in that hour really I could have treated three patients"

Physiotherapist

3.3.1.6 Solutions and resolutions

The ability of SEA to solve problems and resolve awkward issues was generally appreciated. Guidelines for managing a variety of different situations could be discussed and recommended. People could be reassured that they were 'on track' and an agreed direction of travel established, with the opportunity for everyone present to contribute. However, as recognised by Pringle and his colleagues, our participants acknowledged that the short time available could mean that quick, easy or superficial solutions might be adopted. Members also recognised that it was sometimes difficult to be sufficiently honest.

> "I'm not saying that people are shut up, you know, but all you can do is register that you're upset about it and what could be done to stop that problem occurring again. I don't see it as a psychologically supportive arena other than on a fairly superficial level really... I think most of them [significant events] are handled reasonably well, I think perhaps some people might think that they didn't have quite enough time."
>
> Health Visitor

3.3.2   Facilitating SEA

Pringle and his colleagues highlighted a number of important points in relation to the facilitation of the process of SEA. They state, "that successful audit requires a practice leader on audit (not necessarily a doctor); a supportive practice team; an enthusiastic practice manager; trust within the team; re-audit at intervals; explicit agreed standards; protocol development; feedback; and appropriate resources (specifically time, money and staff)... the need to implement change as a consequence of the audit process." We would agree with these points and have identified some additional issues.

3.3.2.1 Rules and guidelines

Participants need a clear set of rules, particularly at the outset. Specifically, managing emotional issues and those affecting absent team members requires agreed ground rules. With an initiative as new and as powerful as SEA, workers feel the need for a defined structure that can provide boundaries for protection, and safety.

As SEA evolves and participants become more comfortable, the structure can change appropriately, with, if necessary, new rules. Our experience has shown that in any event rules need to be revisited and reiterated regularly. Some participants are prepared to take a more pragmatic approach and develop rules with the activity: these are a minority and must be sensitive to the needs of the (possibly less outspoken) majority.

> "it was a forum for disclosure really... It was crucial that people felt that they could say... not only how good everything was, but... 'it's OK to criticise'."
>
> GP

3.3.2.2 Ownership and commitment

Commitment can only be assumed if the participants' need for safety (which the ground rules will have identified) has been addressed. The team has to take responsibility for making it practicable for its members to attend. Full-time workers may find it easier to commit themselves than part-time, job-sharing and lower paid workers, who can be disadvantaged in this respect. This uneven playing field has to be recognised. If the team can address the particular needs of various individuals, providing appropriate cover or in lieu off-duty arrangements, loyalty to SEA meetings can be won.

The evolution of Practice Professional Development Plans (PPDPs) can contribute to formal acknowledgement of SEA for all participants, which will help build corporate ownership.

Commitment also requires judicious selection of topics to ensure continued interest, especially in the early stages (see below).

> "I would (come) if it was relevant... every other Friday is my day off, we get a lot of other meetings, I've got one tomorrow on my day off, and I've got to come into that. So I don't make a habit of coming in unless I feel it's really important..."
>
> Practice Nurse

3.3.2.3 Selection of topics

The needs of all team members must be borne in mind when the SEA agenda is drawn up. If one or more individuals can see little relevance in the topics, it is to be expected that their support will wane. In addition, a sensitive choice of topics is crucial in order to ensure generalisability: the risk of issues becoming personalised, rather than universalised, has to be remembered. Topics which can stimulate the group but which have the potential for resolution which can be dealt with safely are essential.

Other problems with topic selection include the need for awareness of a hot topic becoming cold, items suggested only because no-one else has thought of any ('scraping the barrel') and hidden agendas by one or more individuals. The important issue of individuals' rights to remove proposed topics is addressed separately (see below).

Successful agenda construction (and appropriate modification as the meeting proceeds) is a vital determinant of SEA success and dependent on quality leadership.

> "I think it's got to be handled very carefully, and if you've got to raise issues that might make people feel uncomfortable I think they need to be aware of that before they get involved... I think you've got to have a lot of preparation, rather than just lurching into it without agreement."
>
> Practice Nurse

3.3.2.4 Leadership

Skillful leadership is essential to give confidence and facilitate all these items. Less assertive team members depend upon effective leadership to overcome their hesitancy. The qualities expected from the SEA leadership are extensive, ranging from support and encouragement (before, during and after the actual meetings) (see Management of the process below) through chairing to challenging, summarising, planning and debriefing. This set of qualities is probably not available in any one individual in a practice team, and certainly could seem to rule out rotating the leadership between several people, desirable as this may be.

However, the requirements for leadership are clear and have to be recognised. Once identified, they may be met by the team exploiting its own skill mix, a team building activity that is both contributory to and helped by the process of SEA.

Ensuring a corporate responsibility for leadership is also needed in order to counteract the perennial problem of inequality, both perceived and actual, in the primary care team. Some suggested that the best-placed individual, regardless of personal attributes, to co-ordinate if not provide most of this input is the practice manager. Certainly we were made aware of the difficulties flowing from the often automatic assumption of doctor leadership. Pringle et al also identified leadership as a potential problem in the process of SEA, by stating "leadership is a difficult issue for a general practice team which is said to be non-hierarchical and yet is often led, or apparently led, by doctors or even an individual doctor'.

We encountered gender issues here: participants suggested that female approaches to the challenge of leadership might in general represent a more appropriate model, particularly with regard to ongoing care (see Debriefing).

> "You need positive leadership to put things back in boxes, so people aren't walking away feeling fragile or unresolved or bruised."
>
> Practice Nurse

3.3.2.5 Debriefing

There is an under-recognised need to offer time and support to individuals or groups after SEA meetings. While the ideal is to address and complete all outstanding issues (particularly emotional) within the meeting, it has to be acknowledged that participants are sometimes left with unresolved matters which may be carried on into their next clinical session which might follow immediately. Just as individual learning requires a period of reflection, so too do groups: SEA meetings need to devote attention to this need. Whether individual debriefing should be the responsibility of the leader, the practice manager, a defined group or the whole team, and when and how it is addressed, is less important that the recognition of its need.

> "There is a danger and there is no mechanism for checking out with people at the end of it that they're not really upset or pissed off or whatever... Maybe if just a few of us got together afterwards, you know, people who were involved, specifically involved. But we're so bad at dealing with that sort of stuff. Nobody is used to it really."
>
> GP

3.3.2.6 Censoring and vetting

We would agree that some topics are inappropriate for SEA. We have learnt that individual poor performance needs very sensitive and intimate handling which should not be addressed in an SEA forum. Less professional but no less personal matters (e.g. personal hygiene) are also obviously better dealt with elsewhere. Important as they may be, and indeed needful of attention, there will be confidential (staff health for example), contractual, sex discrimination and other issues which, if the individuals involved do not have the right to strike them from the agenda, can cause severe personal stress and disruption to SEA, if not the practice itself.

> "I would talk to those people involved away from this setting and if I needed to take the issue to the partners, then I'd deal with it in a more sensitive manner, a private manner…"
>
> Practice Manager

3.3.2.7 Management of the process

The whole process of SEA then requires ongoing supervision. The meetings themselves are but part of a continuing developmental spiral, characterised by discussions and preparation leading to SEA which produces actions, review, reflection and reinforcement with perhaps new approaches. All these require active management – management of the practice itself, management of people and management of change. A delicate balance has to be struck between the provision of safety and support, and the stimulation of challenge to improve and ensure quality in all its aspects – a dynamic task, which itself will evolve. Therefore, there has to be adequate opportunity for the team to reflect upon the pace of change, the methods chosen and the progress achieve, and especially the failures – where SEA may be used to audit the process of SEA. Those implementing SEA must present practices with the chance to review, as part of the process. This could be addressed through dedicating a meeting at regular intervals to stocktaking, or to join with one or more other practices to share experiences, or to contribute to a workshop at PCO level. Teams may or may not want to use their own resources with or without imported experts. Possibly the evolving role of clinical governance might facilitate such developments, with its emphasis on joint working at inter- and supra-practice level.

"I think the chairmanship of a particularly negative incident has to be handled very carefully, very carefully, because if they're going to be cosy chats over a cup of tea, you might as well just pack it in. If they are going to be significant, then you might as well make them flipping significant really, and that, I think, takes some skill in the chairmanship. You've got to listen very hard as to how stressed individuals are and you have to be able to allocate responsibility without allocating blame in a personal sense. It sounds very simple, but I think that's a little elusive."

GP

4   CASE STUDY IN PRIMARY CARE

For our follow up study, we used a case study approach to observe a primary care practice over a period of 10 months, employing a Grounded Theory approach to guide both data collection and analysis. The study primary care team was recruited by identifying a team unconnected with the researchers and which, being unexposed to and untrained in SEA, had expressed an interest in being introduced to the technique. The research project was explained and permission granted by members for the study process to take place.

Individuals were recruited after the introductory session, and on the basis of the contribution that they made (or failed to make) to the initial meeting. It was not possible to interview the practice manager at the start of the study as her appointment was being made at the time of commencing the study, but she was included in the post-SEA interviews. We collected data in the following ways;

4.1   Phase 1

Four members of the core team (receptionist, general practitioner, practice nurse, and district nurse) were interviewed at the beginning of the practice's involvement in SEA, and after the initial meeting. The aim of the interview was to explore individuals' expectations of the process of SEA, which was new to them. Interviews were conducted on a one-to-one basis and were tape-recorded.

4.2   Phase 2

Six consecutive SEA meetings were observed over a period of 10 months, with the researcher assuming the role of non-participant observer. Field notes and memos were made both during and after the session, agendas and minutes were retained to supplement the researcher's notes, and a list of attendees was recorded. The aims of this observation phase were to:

- observe SEA in action,
- note the processes involved in reaching and agreeing solutions,
- keep an account of events 'actioned', and
- use the information as baseline from which to inform the post-SEA interviews.

4.3   Phase 3

Following the six observed SEA meetings, the four original core group members were re-interviewed, to examine participants' perceptions in the light of their actual experiences. These interviews were more focused than the first, with the experience of practical issues now able to guide the line of questioning. As before the interviews were conducted on a one-to-one basis, confidentiality was assured and each interview was tape-recorded. In addition, the newly appointed practice manager was interviewed about her experiences of the process and its impact on the practice.

4.4   Phase 4

Finally, a 'negotiated feedback' session was convened in the practice, with the aims of:

- feeding back the findings of the first three phases of the study to the research participants and to the larger group within the practice, and
- checking and clarifying the interpretations with the group.

This session lasted approximately one hour, with 15 minutes of this time devoted to formal feedback. The remaining 45 minutes was spent in discussion, and this session was minuted to provide further data for analysis.

4.5   Analysis of the data

Analysis was carried out in two separate stages. In line with the grounded theory framework used, each interview in the pre-SEA and post-SEA sections of the study was transcribed and then analysed. Data from the negotiated feedback session was used to verify interviewees' perceptions, to check representativeness and to illustrate group perceptions. In addition, the data arising from the six observed meetings was subjected to a content analysis.

4.6   Results

The results of the study are presented under three headings:

1. Preliminary interviews,
2. Observation study, and
3. Post-SEA interviews and feedback session.

4.6.1   Preliminary interviews

Three main findings emerged from these interviews to indicate that participants held a number of expectations of SEA, experienced concerns about the process, and offered suggestions for the successful implementation of the process (Table 2). The notion of SEA was novel to each of the interviewees, although the GP interviewee had been exposed to the concept (but not the reality) of SEA before the groups commenced.

Table 2. Preliminary perceptions of SEA

Expectations of SEA	Concerns about SEA	Suggestions for Implementing SEA
■ Improved relationships	■ Choosing issues	■ Selection of Issues
■ Problem-solving	■ Problem-solving	■ Preparation
■ Outcomes	■ Structural barriers	■ Outcomes
■ Lack of time		■ Leadership
■ Poor outcomes		■ Group Membership
		■ Maintenance of other avenues

4.6.2   Observation study

The SEA meetings were consistently well attended, with between 20 and 22 members of staff attending each meeting (the team consisted of 50 individuals, all of whom had been invited to attend). The meetings, chaired by one of the GP Partners (who volunteered herself for the role), took place approximately every six weeks over a lunch time period. Both surgery and community staff (health visitors, physiotherapists and district nurses) were invited to attend, although attendance at the meetings was entirely voluntary. Lunch was provided on each occasion. Agendas for the current meeting and minutes from the previous meeting were provided to all attendees. The large size of the group caused some concern initially (both to the researcher and to group members), and in an attempt to find the most comfortable and productive group size, three of the SEA sessions split into two groups, whilst the remaining three worked as one group (see discussion).

Twenty-six separate issues were discussed over a period of 10 months at the six SEA meetings. Six of these issues had been presented jointly by individuals from more than one occupational group, one by the District Nurses as a group, and the remainder was presented by one individual. Table 3 indicates that GPs and receptionists most frequently presented events for discussion.

Table 3. Frequency of presentation of significant events by members of different occupational groups

Discipline	Frequency
General practitioners	15 (jointly or singly)
Receptionists	9 (jointly or singly)
District nurses	4 (singly or as a group)
Practice nurse	2 (jointly)
Physiotherapist	2 (singly)

The focus of the significant events and therefore of the meetings was the day-to-day running of the practice and inter-disciplinary communication issues, although some events of a medical nature or of the clinical management of a case were discussed when these were perceived as having a direct bearing on the wider team and could be used to facilitate group learning (Table 4).

Table 4. Nature and frequency of Significant Events

Significant Event	Frequency
Day-to-day administration	10
Diagnosis/clinical management	4
Patients 'hassling' staff	4
Management of clinical emergency	3
Miscommunication	3
Patients rude to staff	1
Extra patients policy	1

As a result of discussing these 26 issues, 62 separate solutions with agreed actions were reached at the meetings. At the end of the period of data collection, 21 of these solutions had been actioned, no feedback was available on 16 of the solutions, 3 had not been actioned after all, 3 were 'on hold', and one was proving complicated and required further discussion. We have grouped the solutions/actions into Pringle's 4 outcomes (Table 5), but feel that a fifth category may be beneficial (see also discussion).

Table 5. Outcomes in terms of Pringle's categories

Category	Frequency
Immediate action	33
Conventional audit	3
Life's like that	2
Congratulations	1
(Further work needed	23) (See discussion below)

4.6.3 Post-SEA interviews and negotiated feedback session

Three findings emerged from the combined results of the post-SEA interviews and the negotiated feedback session. Table 6 indicates that interviewees shared positive perceptions of the benefits of the process ('The Reality of SEA'), that they still had some concerns about the process ('Ongoing Concerns'), and that, in the light of experience, they were able to offer suggestions for the maintenance of the process.

Table 6. The reality of SEA

The reality of SEA	Ongoing concerns
(1) Improved relationships	(1) Shortage of time
(2) Reassurance	(2) Frequency & timing
(3) Feeling of safety	(3) Appropiateness of issues/events
(4) Participation in decision-making	(4) 'Naming and shaming'
(5) Small but important changes	(5) Outcomes difficult to implement and measure
(6) Reaches solutions & actions	(6) Group size
(7) Feeling of working together	(7) Confidentiality and privacy
	(8) Shortage of congratulations
	(9) Individuals dominating meeting

Table 7. Perceptions and experiences post-SEA

Maintaining the process

(1) A healthy and varied agenda
(2) Monitor the overall process every six months
(3) Rotate the day to benefit part-timers
(4) Defer some decisions to Practice Meeting
(5) Summarise actions at end of meeting
(6) Increase number of congratulations
(7) Reconsider venue and group size

4.7   Discussion of results

The study shows that SEA can attract, and continue to attract, primary care workers from a wide variety of backgrounds. Numbers attending remained constant, the activity was well received, all groups actively contributed, and interpersonal relationships, including reassurance, feelings of safety and participation, were all improved.

Participants' expectations of problems being solved, with definite outcomes, were met – indeed 26 issues generated 62 separate solutions with agreed actions. After practising SEA, members felt that solutions had been reached, actions taken and important (even if sometimes small) changes made. But not all outcomes could be implemented, or measured. A substantial number (23) failed to fit comfortably into the standard 4 categories; SEA has a potential capacity to identify areas for quality improvement. In practice, teams sometimes need to ask one or more members to take the opportunity to think more carefully over the particular problem, and bring it back for further discussion and suggestions for improvement.

Concern about the selection of issues remained. Clearly the choice of events is critical: they need to have relevance to the team and engage participants individually, but also to respect personal boundaries and represent material that the team feels able to tackle. Thus leadership – in protecting as well as driving – continues to represent a critical part of successful SEA. Optimal leadership remains unclear. Earlier work by Pringle and his colleagues suggested external facilitation, but this study suggests that it is possible to provide sensitive yet effective leadership from within the practice. However, various leadership issues remained – members were still worried about individuals who dominate, confidentiality, the risk of 'naming and shaming' and achieving and demonstrating outcomes. Discussion at the feedback session concluded that while the leader need not necessarily be a partner, or even a 'senior' partner, the team chose to stay with the GP who volunteered herself for the role. With Clinical Governance contributing further challenges under this heading, the topic of leadership in primary care poses difficult questions beyond, as well as within, the immediate area of SEA.

In general, hierarchical and structural barriers proved less inhibiting than feared, with evidence of receptionists making active contributions, awareness of reassurance and safety and a feeling of participation in all groups. The expectation of improved relationships was fulfilled, but the need to congratulate was underlined. Identifying, acknowledging and celebrating achievements represents one way of moving from traditional attitudes to unacceptable events, system failures and even personal shortcomings, towards mutual support and trust.

Some practical and administrative questions also remain. What is the optimal size of the group? This question will become more important as the imminent generalised roll out of SEA by Clinical Governance leads draws in the full spectrum of practice teams ranging from single-handed practices to very large groups. The present team (a large practice with three branch surgeries, 8 partners plus 1 retained doctor, 13,000 patients and a team of 50 individuals) produced over 20 participants, who experimented with splitting, but eventually decided to meet as one group, convinced that the overall identity and *esprit de corps* outweighed the inevitable difficulties of greater numbers.

What is the relationship between the SEA meetings and partnership and other meetings within the practice? Pressures on time, establishing the optimal frequency and timing of the meetings, determining the agenda and striking the right balance between involving different groups and spreading ownership while maintaining efficient management calls for careful planning and review. Venue and time of the meeting also need to be widely acceptable in order to maintain the process. While there can be no standard answer, these issues need to be decided upon and not underestimated, as they reflect relationships, priorities and underlying philosophies.

The group recommended that a regular six month review of the overall process should take place. But how, by whom and when is another challenge which will need addressing, along with how much information and in what form the team will be prepared to share with clinical governance leads, are issues that will need to be resolved.

5   THE PRISON STUDY

There has been no previous research on SEA in the prison health care unit setting. By observing SEA meetings and evaluating prison health care staffs' attitudes to and understanding of SEA, this study sought to find out:

- the overall impact of SEA
- whether it could be an effective tool in prison health care.

5.1 Participants

SEA was piloted in three prison health care units, two in England and one in Wales. The entire population of eighty-nine members of staff of the health care units were invited to attend the SEA meetings. Of these 78 members were present over the 18 meetings observed. Those present were representative of all the staff groups involved in the health care units; they included 37 nurses, 15 health care officers, 9 doctors, 5 pharmacists, 3 administrators, 3 occupational therapists, a community psychiatric nurse, a member of the board of visitors, a chaplain and a governor. From those attending the initial SEA meetings, a non-probabilistic sample was taken for interview from each prison, to reflect the variety of professions involved so that their different perspectives might be represented in the data. Interviewees included four nurses, three health care officers, two doctors, two pharmacists, two occupational therapists and one community psychiatric nurse.

5.2 Method

Six SEA meetings in each prison were observed, to determine the nature of SEA in-situ. A pro-forma documenting issues, process, solutions and actions was used to make detailed records. The data from these meetings underwent a content analysis to show the profiles of attendance, presenters and contents of the meetings.

Fourteen health care unit staff took part in semi-structured interviews after the first observation and again after the sixth. The interview guide was validated by prior use within primary care. The invitation to participate was by a letter which explained the study in some detail and gave potential participants assurance about the confidentiality of the conversations. The participants were initially interviewed in the health care units in private locations as soon after the first SEA meetings as possible. The interviews were tape recorded and notes were taken. Participants were interviewed again after the sixth SEA observation, to see if their understanding and opinions of SEA had changed.

5.3 Analysis

The use of content analysis to analyse the observational data enabled a clear picture of the content and process of SEA in the health care units to be formed. Issues coded according to type and solutions were categorised, according to Pringle's earlier work.

The verbatim transcripts from the interviews were subject to a qualitative, grounded theory analysis using Atlas.ti software.

5.4 Results and discussion

So what has been the impact of SEA and what is its future in prison health care? The results combine the data from all three prisons.

5.5 Observations

The observation of the 18 SEA meetings showed that 78 members of staff from a variety of professions attended the meetings, with a mean attendance of 10.5 and a range of 6–16 (Box 1). They discussed a range of issues (Box 2); the outcomes were classified, 111 solutions were reached and 72 actions taken (Box 3).

There is evidence from the observations of the meetings that SEA can and does bring about change, that it can be multidisciplinary and encompass a wide range of issues. It is noteworthy that along with clinical issues, items discussed most commonly concerned systems and communication issues, possibly highlighting the need for reform.

5.6 Interviews

The interview analysis revealed the story behind the figures presented in tables 1–3. They combine the results of the initial and follow-up interviews with the negotiated feedback sessions.

5.6.1 Attitudes

Opinions about SEA ranged from the enthusiastic to the cynical. Some reported the pleasure of seeing positive change take place and that SEA made them feel valued. However, most interviewees felt that SEA was a good idea that could not work in HCUs.

BOX 1

"It certainly has proved itself effective in terms of changing nursing practice".

Interview 17

"The movers and shakers amongst us see it as a vehicle for bringing about change ".

Interview 16

"I mean it's (SEA) classic Prison service, terribly cynical about something like that, and I don't want to be because that is part of what some of us are trying to break away from, the automatic cynicism as opposed to considered cynicism, which is hopefully what I'm moving into".

Interview 2

"SEA highlights (the need for) change... but it doesn't actually empower you to implement change".

Interview 19

"I think it's got great potential if we can make it realise its potential...but it is realising it, that's the problem. And there is a defeatist attitude in the prison service; Oh let's not try that because we know it's going to fail".

Interview 17

"Talk doesn't bring change... we need to professionalise the service"

Interview 19

BOX 2

I think it's (SEA) much more supportive, whereas I think staff meetings could be a vehicle for punishment to slag off, or you know, this is going to happen, you will implement. Whereas hopefully this is a decision-making process that everybody is involved in. So rather than it being dictatorial it is sort of led by the group members.

Interview 7

Some staff see it as an opportunity to clear the air, other people use it to highlight their own dilemmas, other people see it as a necessary evil, other people don't know what the hell it's all about.

Interview 1

It is just an ongoing problem, it is the team thing, because we just don't work as a team, which is very sad.

Interview 10

5.6.2 Understanding

Interviewees thought that other staff did not understand what SEA was about and that in some prisons SEA had lost its format. It was perceived simply as a safe place for a structured discussion; while this was valued, it lacked the dynamic of SEA. The perception remained that it was a management tool. Although solutions to problems were being found they were often not implemented and SEA had generally not made an impact on the day-to-day life of the staff. The ability to discuss matters with colleagues was valued although it was not generally felt that this had led to team-building; any team-spirit generated in the meetings was not being carried through in the units. As these misunderstandings may be partly the result of individuals missing the introductory sessions due to shift working, a more thorough introduction to SEA may be needed which accounts for this problem.

BOX 3

You know sometimes it's (the issue) been dealt with properly and at other times things slip back.

Interview 17

There is a feeling that it doesn't matter what the rank and file do, management implement the changes they want.

Interview 17

5.6.3 Effectiveness

Where changes were acknowledged it was generally believed that these would not be sustained and could only have impact on health care issues, so that any problems that overlapped with the rest of the prison were insoluble by the team. This was because decision making was perceived to occur elsewhere in the prison i.e. by governors. Feedback of the outcomes of the meetings was generally poor and appeared to rely on minutes, which most people did not read.

5.6.4 Leadership

Leadership was an issue. It was felt some training would be helpful and that having non-managers as leaders would make SEA more acceptable. The term 'significant event' was misleading to some who interpreted it as meaning major event eg. Suicide.

> I don't think the Chair necessarily has to be the most senior person present. There does need to be someone who is comfortable with the role.
>
> Interview 2

5.6.5 Attendance

Another concern was the poor attendance at the meetings. Various ideas were put forward to improve this, from making attendance compulsory to providing a lunch or paying people to attend. In prisons where SEA was held on training afternoons this was not thought to be helpful as there were too many conflicting demands on staff time, it was strongly felt that SEA needed dedicated time. The people who attended the meetings tended to reflect the divisions within the staff, eg mainly 'day care' or managers, so SEA was to some extent seen by health care unit staff as a meeting for 'us or them'.

The follow-up interviews revealed a small positive shift in attitudes. There was a group of staff in each prison who valued and understood the potential of SEA. However, for the majority it seems that it was just another meeting.

6   CONCLUSIONS

Our preliminary study in primary care builds on the earlier work by Pringle and others. By using a different methodology and a different sample, we successfully confirmed findings of previous research, and extended our knowledge of the subject. Many of the benefits of SEA, such as its ability to stimulate clinical audit and needs assessment, to inform commissioning and improve quality, have been well documented. In terms of the process, it can be seen that SEA represents a powerful team-building experience for primary care team members, capable of involving all members in a multidisciplinary approach and creating better morale. All members can appreciate the individual benefits along with the better communication, improved mutual understanding, happier work environment and the resulting enhanced patient care. These are important contributions to the well functioning primary care team demanded by today's NHS.

However, there are substantial difficulties, not previously documented, which not only can prevent the successful implementation of SEA but which can alienate individuals and cause damage to teams. Members fear exposure, find it difficult to step out of role, worry about causing offence (especially to GPs who may be their employers) and need sensitive encouragement based upon an awareness of these various anxieties. However, by establishing clear rules, ensuring general ownership, carefully selecting the right topics and using good leadership skills, allowing for proper support and protecting individuals, SEA may be implemented successfully.

Our study has shown that teams and their members have derived many personal, professional and corporate benefits from SEA. The new emphasis upon clinical governance requires structures and processes which can create and sustain a framework for individual professionals and teams to respond to the new agenda for quality improvement. Our research leaves us in no doubt that SEA represents a crucially important tool for primary care teams. As with all new tools, both training and support are needed to ensure optimal use and indeed prevent damage. However, by following our suggestions for facilitating the process, we believe teams will be able to introduce and maintain SEA as a powerful opportunity to strengthen teamwork, enhance quality and improve patient care, its benefits far outweighing its disadvantages.

The *case study in primary care* helps us to reach further conclusions. By assessing the expectations of members of a primary care team before undertaking SEA, observing them pursuing the activity and interviewing them with a negotiated feedback session after ten months, we have had the opportunity to assess the impact of SEA, particularly in terms of the benefits achieved as seen by the participants. Confirming earlier research, the case study shows that the overall experience was found to be useful in team building, and generating worthwhile improvements in patient care, so that SEA was well supported. But fears concerning personal blaming, appropriateness of issues and events, difficulty at times in implementing and measuring outcomes, and worries about confidentiality and privacy issues, as well as continuing questions on administrative aspects of the activity remain. However, convinced of its benefits, the team has now adopted SEA as an integral part of its life and work. Participants made some practical suggestions for maintaining the process to include part-timers, reinforced certain aspects of SEA (particularly the need to summarise action points) and stressed the need to find cause for congratulation.

Finally, our *prison study* demonstrates that SEA has the potential to bring about change in prison health care. It has been shown to be an effective tool; however the challenge of whether it will be well used lies in the attitudes and understanding of health care staff. A comprehensive introduction to SEA is therefore vital. There was a feeling overall that a lot of change was underway in prison health care and that SEA was part of an evolving system. SEA needs to be presented as a tool for managing change as well as monitoring events. It can enhance staff development and be a supportive, professional, multidisciplinary tool, which as part of clinical governance, can help to enable change in a positive way. If SEA is to succeed it requires acceptance throughout the prison hierarchy and to be introduced to the health care staff within the broader context of clinical governance.

7   IS THERE EVIDENCE THAT SEA FACILITATES CLINICAL GOVERNANCE?

Clinical governance leads seem to value SEA as a focus for clinical governance activity. What is it about SEA that makes it such a useful tool in meeting the challenges posed by clinical governance? Much of the direction of development of clinical governance is emerging from the NHS Clinical Governance Support Team (CGST) in Leicester. The CGST highlight the importance of five cornerstones of clinical governance, namely *systems awareness, teamwork, communication, ownership* and *leadership*. We suggest that SEA addresses all five cornerstone of clinical governance in a very practical way.

7.1   Systems awareness

SEA takes a "no-blame" approach, looking at *what is wrong, not who is wrong*". Issues are raised from SEA meetings which are often quite complex. These cannot always be solved during the hour-long meeting, but a small team is identified to work through the problem and come to the next meeting with suggestions for improving the system. A mistake with repeat prescribing in a general practice may lead to an overhaul of the repeat prescribing system. The small group nominated to undertake the task would include the practice manager, receptionist, doctor and possibly dispenser. They would bring back a draft proposal to be discussed and supported by the larger group.

7.2   Teamwork

Patients hardly ever have an experience of health care involving only one person or profession. In order to see the GP, the receptionist makes an appointment. Long-term care of people with diabetes takes place in the main in general practice. Although the practice nurse is increasingly becoming the key worker, the general practitioner has a critical role, as does the chiropodist, dietician and diabetes specialist nurse in certain circumstances. From the patient's viewpoint, their support team may change over time, but the practice nurse will probably remain the key point of contact. At times, the team will cross the traditional boundaries between primary and secondary care. SEA helps team members to understand more about the role of others, and to value their contribution. For many years, GPs have tried to sort out their appointment systems. They only have to ask the receptionists for their input, and immediate progress is made!

7.3　Communication

Many significant events arise due to lack of communication. Getting teams into a room on a regular basis to discuss adverse events will not only highlight communication deficits, but also begin to improve the situation. Communication between organisations is even more of a problem. Inviting visitors to contribute on certain agenda items at the SEA meeting not only helps to get better solutions, but also helps those involved to see things from the perspective of others. The elderly patient, who has been waiting for months for their appointment for the Pain Clinic, is understandably devastated when the ambulance fails to pick him up. The consequences for the patient, the practice and the hospital clinic are immeasurable, and the ambulance staff should be involved in the discussions to prevent a similar event from happening again.

7.4　Ownership

With simpler problems, the team will be involved in generating the solution during the meeting, ensuring ownership of those present. The meetings are minuted and circulated to the whole team, but those present will have a higher level of ownership. With more complex problems, a small group will be delegated to come up with draft proposals for the next meeting, when the wider team will adapt and support the recommendations. SEA meetings are often the first opportunity for people, who are traditionally not in positions of decision-making, to shape solutions.

Early on, receptionists and secretaries appreciate this new feeling of influence. Conversely, traditional decision-makers, such as doctors and senior managers feel uncomfortable, yet should be appreciated of the better solutions, as well as their wider ownership.

7.5 Leadership

The success of SEA meetings depends on good facilitation and leadership. As SEA becomes more widely adopted, there will be a need to develop leaders. The traditional leaders are not necessarily the best facilitators of SEA. In a hospital unit, where a consultant started as chairman, the meeting were well attended by doctors and only a few nurses. The lead was changed to a nurse manager, and the meeting immediately became more popular, more multidisciplinary and more effective. A similar switch from doctor to nurse had an identically beneficial effect on another ward. In a general practice, a new female partner, with a quietly efficient manner proved an excellent leader of the SEA meetings in a general practice comprising a number of powerful doctor personalities, with little history of teamwork.

As well as being a force for quality improvement, there is evidence that SEA is also an important part of multi-professional continuing professional development. It identifies learning needs as well as being a means of team learning, linking to individual learning portfolios and also the revalidation process. There is also the mutual support element, which is crucial at a time of rising levels of stress, encouraging a feeling of looking out for each other. Both clinical governance and SEA focus on people, both patients and professionals. They are both about improving care and learning together. SEA provides an important link between learning and quality improvement in a multi-professional setting.

Chapter 8

A case study of Significant Event Audit: congratulations

'First, and most importantly, significant event auditing can identify good practice. How often do we congratulate our colleagues on good care? A patient attended the nurse for a 'flu vaccination. The nurse noticed that the patient was pale and a little breathless. She took a full blood count that showed a chronic leukaemia. The team recognises and congratulates her on her initiative.'

Pringle, 2000: 111–112

1   INTRODUCTION

A significant event audit meeting should result in at least one outcome (see chapter 2), although as we have indicated it is often the case that any one issue addressed at a meeting will generate a range of solutions which can fit comfortably into a number of different categories. According to Pringle and his colleagues there are four different outcome categories, the first of which he has termed 'Congratulations'. To us this is one of the most important categories and indeed is one of the great strengths of SEA. In an environment like the NHS praise for a job well done is often in extremely short supply. Often care and treatment is exemplary and we would argue that even in the worst or most difficult situation, teams can find examples of excellent practice, which should be acknowledged and commended. SEA helps to formalise this acknowledgement and commendation.

The purpose of this chapter is to present a short case study to illustrate the category comprising 'congratulations'. The case study is drawn from a real life situation in a primary care setting and arose with one of the primary care teams that participated in our research (see chapter 7) and that we were fortunate enough to observe. We have used a little artistic licence when recounting this story so that we can protect the identities of the individuals and teams involved in the incident, and can better illuminate the messages that we feel are important to highlight. The chapter is divided into four sections:

■ The team's history with SEA,
■ The case presented,
■ The solutions generated by the team, and
■ The Outcome categories.

We will conclude the chapter by drawing together the main lessons that the team learnt in terms of developing SEA as a result of collectively reflecting on this particular case.

2   THE TEAM'S HISTORY WITH SEA

This was a large practice in a busy market town. The primary care team was made up of 7 GPs (plus one retainer), 5 receptionists, 6 administrative staff, 2 practice nurses and a practice manager. The core team was complemented by a group of district nurses, health visitors and midwives, plus a physiotherapist who held regular clinics at the surgery. The community psychiatric nurse and a representative from social services visited the practice on a regular basis and attended multidisciplinary case meetings as and when they needed to. This wider team was invited to attend the SEA meetings.

The team worked in a training and research practice and all the clinical staff were comfortable with the notion of Continuing Professional Development, external review and so on. Clinical Governance as a theoretical concept was beginning to rear its head, and the partners felt that it was important to 'keep ahead of the game'. As a result of the interests held by many of the GPs and nursing staff in education, ongoing professional development and clinical audit, SEA seemed like the next logical step for the practice. It must be said that this enthusiasm for SEA was not shared by all members of the team, particularly by the administrative and reception staff, who felt that the meetings would simply provide an opportunity for the GPs to 'tell them off' in front of their colleagues. Similar concerns were expressed by other members of the group. The team itself was going through quite a difficult phase and was viewed by some as unnecessarily hierarchical. However, the 'enthusiasts' persevered and invited a local 'expert' (the first author) along to provide further information about the technique to the whole team (including colleagues from the community).

The presentation took the form of a short overview of the method and aims of SEA, some small group work (having a go at doing it) and wider discussion and debriefing. Although the session did not entirely convince the sceptics, it did provide some comfort to them and re-affirmed the non-judgmental ethos of the approach. All agreed to 'give it a go'. Meetings were scheduled for once every six weeks. These took place at lunch time, replaced an already existing uni-professional meeting and were very well supported with an average of 22 people attending every meeting over the first 10 months. A drug company provided lunch in exchange for access to the GPs. A female junior partner ('Susan') was nominated to chair the meetings. Susan and the practice manager ('Sarah') met prior to the meeting to choose items for the agenda. A typed agenda and minutes from the previous meeting was sent to all attendees prior to the meeting. The case below was presented at the second meeting of the SEA group.

3   THE CASE PRESENTED

One of the GPs ('Simon') presented a case that had gone very well. The case involved Simon himself, one of the practice nurses and one of the receptionists. The main points are presented below:

> At 10.10am on a busy Monday morning, a middle-aged man walked into the reception area with his wife. Although there were two receptionists on duty, one was booking patients in for their appointments and the other was answering telephone calls. There was a queue of about six patients (some becoming slightly irate at the delay) waiting to see the receptionist.

The receptionist who had been taking the telephone calls noticed that the man who had recently arrived actually looked quite unwell (pale, frightened, fighting for breath and clammy). She called the gentleman to the front of the queue, who stated that he had suddenly felt very unwell while he had been out walking with his wife (they happened to be passing the surgery) and had called in to the surgery on the off-chance of seeing a doctor. The receptionist quickly noted that all the GPs were in mid-consultation, having patients with them, but noticed that a woman was just leaving the practice nurses' treatment room. The receptionist escorted the gentleman and his wife around to the treatment room.

On arrival at the treatment room the man collapsed. The nurse managed to get him on to an examination couch, checked his airway and vital signs. The following sequence of events rapidly unfolded:

- the nurse called the nearest doctor ('Simon')
- the nurse had done all the correct things before Simon arrived
- the receptionist phoned an ambulance (off her own bat) that arrived within 7 minutes
- the wife informed the nurse that her husband had swallowed a bee
- the wife was present in the treatment room throughout the period of treatment, and the nurse kept her calm and well informed on Simon's arrival
- the man left in the ambulance when his condition had stabilised
- all three staff met later in the day over coffee for a quick debrief and check that everyone was feeling OK
- the surgery later phoned the hospital to check on his progress
- the man made a full recovery
- he/his wife later phoned to thank the surgery for their prompt action that had almost certainly saved his life.

Simon (in consultation with the practice nurse and the receptionist) brought this particular event to the meeting as a Significant Event because it was felt that:

- The event demonstrated quick reactions and excellent teamwork which deserved praise and acknowledgement
- It provided a vehicle for sharing good practice and for wider learning
- It highlighted an unmet training need within the practice.

There were a few immediate changes that could be implemented to make sure that a similar incident in the future could run even more smoothly.

Discussion of the significant event offered the opportunity for support and catharsis for the staff involved in this dramatic incident.

The group discussed the significant event for approximately 25 minutes, and arrived at a number of solutions (see below). In addition, group members were generous in their praise for the way in which the incident had been handled from the patient's first arrival in the surgery to his leaving the premises in an ambulance.

4   THE SOLUTIONS GENERATED

As is common with a complex case like this, the team generated a number of solutions after a detailed analysis of this case. These were:

- The receptionist was highly praised for her accurate analysis of the urgency of the patient's condition, for her correct response in getting the patient to the treatment room immediately, for contacting the ambulance service without delay, and for her calm and reassuring manner with the patient and his wife.
- The practice nurse was highly praised for her clinical management of the patient prior to Simon's arrival, and for her calm, confident and reassuring manner with the patient and his wife.
- The ambulance service was praised (in their absence) for their speedy arrival.

The practice nurse identified some of the logistical issues that had made things go so well – the movable examination couch, monitoring equipment, emergency drugs and equipment.

However she also identified some improvements that could be made to the resuscitation room and to the tray of equipment.

One of the doctors drew attention to new guidelines on resuscitation that had recently been produced by the Department of Health – all clinical staff were to receive a copy of these and discuss any arising issues at the subsequent SEA meeting.

Reception staff in particular highlighted their need for training in Basic Life Support. One of the partners agreed to explore the possibility of establishing Basic Life Support training for all staff at the surgery. It was decided that this would become an annual event.

5   OUTCOME CATEGORIES

The primary outcome for this significant event was congratulations, although analysis of the case also highlighted a training need, identified new guidelines and informed some minor alterations to the resuscitation room and equipment.

6   CONCLUSIONS

In addition to reaching a number of practical solutions, reflection on this particular case made the team aware of a wider range of issues, including:

- Because some members of the team were reluctant and anxious about SEA, it was important to 'manage' the agenda and ensure that a fair balance of positive items were placed on the agenda. It was particularly important to highlight good examples of team working (a special aspect of SEA is how it can allow teams to praise themselves for their own achievements).
- Getting people on board was made easier by the provision of a social aspect to the meetings – these were held in a relaxed environment over lunch that was provided as an 'incentive' for busy professionals.
- Discussion of the event was comforting to members of the team who felt reassured that their colleagues coped so well in a crisis situation. They knew that they could rely on each other.
- Debriefing immediately after the event was important – discussion of such an event should not be postponed to the next meeting but needs to be aired soon after the incident has occurred.
- The role of leader is a particularly important one with an initially reluctant team. The female GP who led this group provided a safe, secure, non-judgmental environment for the whole team to work within.

■ Group size was an issue for this team. Organisational psychology literature suggests that teams work best with 8–12 members, and several attempts were made with this primary care team to split them into two groups of 10–12 people (coming together for feedback at the end) but this did not work well for this particular group; they wanted to work as one large team.

SEA can help teams to identify training needs that are truly relevant and appropriate to the needs of the individuals within the team.

Even where there is excellent care, there are always opportunities to improve.

Chapter 9

A case study of Significant Event Audit: immediate action

'Some events clearly expose systematic weaknesses in the care of the practice. A patient has a stroke and the last entry in the notes reveals a very high blood pressure, but the patient did not attend for review. This is acknowledged to be both a serious and a common problem. The practice agrees to alter its recall system to allow such patients to be followed up if they fail to attend.'

Pringle et al, 1995: 24

1   INTRODUCTION

We have seen that a significant event audit meeting should results in at least one outcome (chapter 2), although we have already mentioned that it is often the case that any one significant event will generate a range of solutions that can fit into a number of different categories. The second of Pringle's outcome categories has been termed 'Immediate Action'.

The purpose of this chapter is to present a short case study to illustrate the category comprising 'immediate action'. The case study is drawn from a real life situation in a primary care setting and also arose with one of the primary care teams that participated in our research (see chapter 7). As before, we have used a little artistic licence when recounting this story so that we can protect the identities of the individuals and teams involved in the incident, and can illuminate the message that we wish the reader to go away with. The chapter is divided into four sections:

1. The team's history with SEA,

2. The case presented,

3. The solutions generated by the team, and

4. The outcome categories.

We will conclude by drawing together the main lessons that the participating practice learnt as a result of collectively reflecting on this particular case, in terms of developing SEA within the team.

2   THE TEAM'S HISTORY WITH SEA

This primary care team consisted of four GP principals, four administrative staff, three receptionists, a practice nurse and a practice manager. In addition, SEA meetings were open to the health visiting, midwifery and district nursing teams who regularly accepted the invitation to attend the SEA meeting.

One of the partners had initially developed an interest in the use of SEA within the practice following his attendance at a regional study day on the process. The concept was met with little reluctance from team members. After some gentle persuasion with the rest of the team and following a short training session, the meetings took place once a month at lunch times.

The team was fortunate that the time for the SEA meetings was protected and that the building was closed to patients during the hour-long lunch time session. Group participants brought their own packed lunches. The meetings were chaired by 'Mark', the GP partner who originally expressed an interest in the process. Mark was the first to admit that that his rise to 'group facilitator' was more by a process of default than design! Mark in his role as group chairman also selected the items for each meetings agenda from the 'SEA book'. The process of choosing issues for discussion at the meetings was shared between Mark and 'Mary', the practice manager a day or so prior to the meeting. A typed agenda with short minutes of the previous meeting was then circulated to all attendees. On average SEA meetings in this practice were attended by 8 members of the primary care and wider community team.

The case that we have chosen to present was discussed at the fourth meeting of this group.

3   THE CASE PRESENTED

A particularly emotive and sensitive case for discussion was brought to the meeting by Mary, the practice manager. Mary had been alerted to the incident by one of the receptionists who had been on duty at the time of the incident and felt in a stronger position than the receptionist to present the event in front of the team. As is traditional with SEA, a brief history of the case was presented to the group. In presenting, Mary was careful to refer to the patient's case notes on her lap and regularly checked facts with the reception staff and the GP who were involved with the incident. Briefly the case involved the following:

> A young woman came to visit her doctor for what should have been a regular antenatal check-up at twelve weeks of pregnancy. This was the woman's first pregnancy and was very welcome. Sadly, the woman had miscarried one week prior to this routine appointment. Living in a small and tight knit community, the reception staff (who knew the patient and her family on a social basis) were aware of the miscarriage, but the GP was not aware of the events and assumed that the woman was still attending for her antenatal check.
>
> At the start of the consultation, the GP, Michael congratulated the woman on how well she looked, asked after the health of the baby, and checked that she was attending for her routine antenatal check-up. It was immediately clear to the patient that her family doctor was not aware of her miscarriage. The patient was understandably distraught, and realising his error, the GP felt awkward and embarrassed. The consultation continued but both patient and GP felt uncomfortable and dissatisfied. After surgery, Michael spoke to the patient's health visitor, the reception staff and the practice manager about his horror at what had happened. For her part, after reflecting on the incident over night, the patient contacted the practice manager to express her anger and dissatisfaction at the 'shoddy and insensitive' way that she felt she had been treated by the surgery. Mary and the GP apologised to the patient on the telephone, before composing a letter of apology and explanation to the patient and her partner.

Mary and Mark (in consultation with the GP and the receptionist) decided to bring this issue as a Significant Event because:

- It provided a vehicle for wider learning
- It involved poor communication, a feature of life in a busy practice
- There were immediate changes that could be made to prevent a re-occurrence of the incident
- Discussion of the significant event offered the opportunity for support and catharsis for the staff involved in the incident.

The group discussed the significant event for approximately 15 minutes, and arrived at a number of solutions (see below). In addition, group members were aware that Michael was feeling that he had let both the patient and the team down, and were particularly conscious to support the way that he handled the situation once it became apparent that a mistake had occurred. There was a strong feeling of 'there for the Grace of God'. Everyone in the team was reminded of the sometimes sensitive issues and vulnerable people that they work with on a day-to-day basis, and of the need to remain sensitive and perceptive to the needs of their patients, even in their busy surgery.

4   THE SOLUTIONS GENERATED

It was agreed by all present that every effort must be made by the collective group to prevent this type of distressing mis-communication from occurring in the future. The following solutions were suggested and agreed by all:

- The GPs and other clinical staff were reminded that they should not pre-judge the patient's needs at the beginning of the consultation. The group discussed various ways that they might begin the session so that the patient would have an opportunity to disclose any changes in his/her condition or circumstances. It was felt that a more open 'what can I do for you today?' could be more sensitive than 'so you've come for your 12-week check?' All clinical staff agreed to try these new openings and report back to the subsequent SEA meeting.
- It was agreed that once the surgery received notification of a patient's miscarriage, the reception staff would put a visible note in a prominent position on the patient's notes and computer records to alert the GP, health visitor or practice nurse to the changed circumstances.

- In addition, it was agreed that reception staff would record the miscarriage on the surgery white-board, which could only be accessed by and visible to members of the primary care team and which was already in use to alert the team to urgent issues.
- All patients who suffered a miscarriage were to be sent a letter from the surgery as a matter of routine and invited to make an appointment with the GP, midwife or Health Visitor for a physical check-up and to provide psychological support. In addition, it was suggested that patients would be given a booklet on miscarriage to support and reassure them through this difficult period.

Finally all staff acknowledged that this error, although very distressing for the patient and the GP involved, could happen to any member of the team, and several people shared similar incidences or 'near misses' with Michael.

5   OUTCOME CATEGORIES

All of these proposed solutions fell into Pringle's category of 'immediate action' as it was agreed at the SEA meeting that these solutions would take immediate effect to prevent a similar incident at the practice. The issue was revisited as a matter of routine at the subsequent SEA meeting to check that the new systems for recording and disseminating this type information were in place.

6   CONCLUSIONS

In addition to reaching a number of practical solutions, reflection on this particular case made the team aware of a wider range of issues including:

- Even sensitive and embarrassing issues can be addressed in SEA if the team is strong and supportive and adopts a no-blame culture.
- It is permissible for groups of individuals to band together to present a case, particularly if the individual presenter is likely to feel vulnerable or disenfranchised.

- It is important to have 'close to hand' all the facts and figures relevant to the particular case under discussion as it is likely that these will be referred to during the meeting.
- The solutions to this issue were incredibly simple and did not involve spending large sums of practice money, but had the potential to contribute significantly to the smoother running of life in the practice.
- The solutions were "systems" based. No one individual or group of individuals was held accountable for the error that had occurred.
- Whilst recognising the distress that had been caused to the patient, the individual clinician was supported in his handling of a difficult situation.

Chapter 10

A case study of Significant Event Audit: further work is called for

'Investigate the situation further. This may take the form of getting advice from another doctor, performing a literature review, seeking out a guideline, or talking to the patient and the family. Precipitate action in response to an event may be unwise; failing to reflect on what may have happened is equally unwise. This link between events and the educational needs of individuals and the whole team is, in our experience, very powerful.'

Pringle, 2000: 112

1   INTRODUCTION

Pringle's termed his third category of outcomes as 'Further Work' (see chapter 2). One of the potential difficulties of SEA is the possibility of dealing with events in a superficial manner because of shortage of time, pressure to come up with a solution or lack of appropriate data. In the course of our observation studies, we have certainly come across one or two events that could have been handled more effectively if the team had had more time to consider the range of solutions or access to further data. Similarly, we have observed teams take an event away for further work, and come back with creative and/or evidence-based solutions. This initially may require some courage, in a busy environment that often demands speedy interventions. We feel that it is entirely appropriate that discussion of a significant event can generate further legitimate work in the form of conventional audits, small group work, protocol developments, policy changes, literature reviews, and so on.

As Pringle rightly indicates, a training programme that is developed in response to the genuine requirements of the team (as highlighted during SEA) must be preferable to the ad hoc selection of individually interesting courses or study days. We have encountered team who develop their whole clinical governance agenda on the basis of the outcomes of their SEA meetings in terms of risk management and ongoing professional development for the team members.

In this chapter we will present a brief case study to illustrate the category of 'further work'. As usual the real-life case has been selected from one of the teams that we were able to observe as part of our research program. This particularly case study is drawn from the secondary care setting. As indicated in the earlier chapters, we have also altered aspects of this story so that we can protect the identities of the team, and the individuals involved.

The chapter is presented in four different sections:

1. The team's history with SEA,
2. The case presented
3. The solutions generated by the team, and
4. The outcome categories.

To conclude the chapter, we will try to draw together the wider lessons that this team learnt about the development of SEA within this environment, as a result of reflecting on this particular case.

2   THE TEAM'S HISTORY WITH SEA

This large team worked in the busy Emergency Department (ED) of a large District General Hospital. SEA was first introduced to the team by one of the ED consultants ('David') who was aware that a colleague of his had successfully introduced the technique on one of the neighbouring high-risk wards. David was young, progressive and very keen to promote and encourage multi-disciplinary team working on the ED. The clinical team members were all highly skilled, used to working in a highly charged environment and used to depending on each other for support and appropriate back-up every working day. No team member expressed any serious reservations at David's suggestion to introduce SEA on a regular basis.

The SEA meetings were scheduled to take place every 4-6 weeks in a large meeting room. All members of the ED were invited to attend (including portering staff and clerical staff) as well as allied services like radiography and physiotherapy. Because of his position in the team and because he was the person to introduce SEA, David opted to chair the SEA meetings in the absence of others volunteering for the role. However after about 6 months, when it became clear that the majority of regular attendees were junior medical staff and a handful of senior nursing staff, David suggested that it might be appropriate to change the leader. The senior nurse ('Dawn') was an enthusiastic supporter of SEA, having attended all the ED meetings since the technique was introduced, and having actively encouraged the nursing staff to participate and contribute. Dawn agreed to lead the meeting, and under her chairmanship (David continued to attend in the capacity of group member), the meetings continued to flourish and drew a larger and more multidisciplinary team.

The 'significant events' book was held in a central spot in the department that was accessible to all staff but safe from the prying eyes of patients, their relatives and the general public. Members of staff were encouraged to write events in the book and shortly prior to the meeting, Dawn and David met to select items for the agenda. Agendas and minutes were sent to all staff attending the meeting and posted in the common room for staff (e.g. those on night duty) who were unable to attend. Because of the sometimes volatile nature of work on the ED, space was kept free to enable the inclusion of 'hot topics' during the meeting.

The case selected for presentation in this case study was discussed at the sixth SEA meeting of the team.

3 THE CASE PRESENTED

The case was presented by 'Dorothy', one of the staff nurses in the ED, in conjunction with nursing and medical colleagues who were familiar with the incident. Dorothy described the main points of the case as follows:

At 3.30 in the morning, Dorothy took a phone call from Ambulance Control Headquarters, who were alerting the ED to the imminent arrival of up to five trauma victims from a serious road traffic accident. The caller at Ambulance Control described how several ambulances and paramedics were at the scene of the accident, and would begin to ferry the seriously injured victims to the hospital (15 miles away) within the next 10–15 minutes.

As all senior medical staff were off duty by the stage that the call had been received and the nursing staff were already occupied with other patients, Dorothy wondered whether it was appropriate for her to make the judgement as to whether or not the current staffing could cope with the incoming patients. Dorothy was an experienced staff nurse. There was no one more senior or more experienced for Dorothy to speak with (the junior medical staff had just begun their rotation on the ED). She was becoming conscious that time was ticking away, and that the first patients would be due to arrive at any time. Before making a decision, Dorothy thought that she would check that she had heard properly from the Ambulance Control, and after spending five minutes trying to contact them, she eventually got through to them. However Ambulance Control had not heard any more from the crew, and could not provide any more up to date information. Dorothy decided to call in the Trauma Team, all of whom arrived at the hospital within 15 minutes.

When the ambulance, ferrying the accident victims, arrived at the ED, Dorothy felt slightly foolish when one person with what transpired to be a broken ankle, emerged from the vehicle. The gentleman was accompanied by two friends, both of whom were sporting minor cuts and bruises. Although all the ED staff were relieved that no one was seriously injured in the accident, one or two members of the Trauma Team complained that they had been called to attend the department for no legitimate reason. Members of the Trauma Team went home, as Dorothy and her colleagues continued to treat the patients in the department. In addition, Dorothy spoke briefly to the paramedics (who had arrived with the patients) about the miscommunication. The paramedics did not understand how Ambulance Control had managed to convey the incorrect message and agreed to speak to them to clarify the importance of conveying the correct message to the receiving ED.

Dorothy (in consultation with the medical and nursing teams) brought this particular event to the meeting as a Significant Event because it was felt that:

- It provided a vehicle for wider learning
- It highlighted the possibility of a policy change or at least the clarification of a policy issue within the department.
- The event demonstrated quick reactions which deserved praise and acknowledgement.
- Discussion of the significant event offered the opportunity for support and catharsis for the staff involved in the incident .

The group discussed the significant event for approximately 15 minutes, and arrived at a number of solutions (see below). In addition, all group members were generous in their praise for the way in which Dorothy had handled the incident in the absence of clear information from Ambulance Control.

4   THE SOLUTIONS GENERATED

A number of solutions were generated by the team in response to this particular case. They were:

- David (the consultant) would seek an early meeting with Chief of the Ambulance Service, in order to clarify issues (and decide on solutions) around occasionally apparent difficulties with communication. [The outcome of that meeting – they actually bought mobile phones for the ambulance crews so that they could speak directly to the ED team from the 'field'– a fantastic but so simple solution!]
- It was agreed that David, Dorothy, a member from Ambulance Control, and a paramedic would set up a small working group to consider the need for a clearer protocol for staff on the ED to follow in the future.Dawn (the senior nurse and group facilitator) would look into the possibility of installing another dedicated line between the ED and Ambulance Control, as it was sometimes difficult to access them at busy times.

- Dawn would write to the Ambulance Service and invite them to send a representative to the SEA meeting on a regular basis, but particularly at the next meeting when they could feed back on progress that had been made in trying to address this case.

5   THE OUTCOME CATEGORIES

Most of the solutions to this particular case fell into Pringle's category of Further Work, although one of the senior medical staff took the opportunity to congratulate the nursing staff on the increasing number of appropriate trauma calls that they had made independently. In addition, Dorothy was reassured that she had made the correct decision with the amount of information that she had received.

6   CONCLUSIONS

In addition to reaching some practical solutions, reflection on this particular issue served to make the team aware of some wider issues that impacted on the SEA meetings. These included:

- The ED had a large core team that was dependent on a wider group, including the Ambulance and Fire Services, Portering Services, Catering Services, Radiography and Physiotherapy. For the effective running of the meetings, it was agreed that there was a need to invite representatives from these key departments to the meetings and to send them copies of minutes and agendas in case of absences.

- Because of the nature of work in secondary care, it was considered necessary to make special arrangements to accommodate shift changes and the team were considering the most appropriate way of keeping the whole team up-to-date whilst keeping the SEA group to a manageable size and running meetings at a time in the day when senior members of staff could temporarily leave the department.

- The change of leadership had an important impact on the SEA meetings in terms of the way in which ownership amongst the nursing staff changed, when the leadership role shifted to the senior nurse. Although a natural leader and an egalitarian individual, the consultant (by virtue of his position in the hierarchy) may have intimidated some of the junior medical and nursing staff members. Contributions from all junior and non-clinical staff flourished under the nurse's leadership, who enjoyed the respect of the senior medical and management personnel of the hospital.

■ After about six months, the ED team decided to change of name from the 'SEA Meeting' to the 'ED Open Meeting' as some members of the team felt that the term 'significant' implied that events should have dramatic or negative connotations. Indeed in secondary care, the use of the word may have reminded people of case conferences and postmortems.

■ One of the nurses pointed out that almost everything that the staff on the ED deal with as part of their day-to-day work could be termed 'significant'. It was particularly important then, in a setting such as this, to clarify the role and boundaries around SEA so that group members knew how to use the meetings properly.

Chapter 11

A case study of Significant Event Audit: life's like that

'The last outcome from our discussions is to agree that there are no lessons to be learnt. The case illustrates normal primary [or other] care, and there are no particular features to be discussed in depth. These are the most common cases but they cannot necessarily be identified in advance.'

Pringle, 2000: 112 *(comment in brackets added)*

1   INTRODUCTION

Pringle called his fourth and final outcome category 'Life's Like That' (chapter 2). We feel that this is a particularly important category in a work setting that is often full of risks and unpredictable variables. It is clear that many risks can be contained and minimised, and indeed one of the core principles of clinical governance is the development of systematic structures and systems that can make the work of health care safer and less risky. However, we must also recognise that taking risks is an important part of progress and that it is not possible or desirable to manage and control all aspects of life, working or otherwise. Sometimes when events are outside of our control we need to be able to accept that events are not always controllable and to move on. This is Pringle's 'Life's Like That' category. It should be noted that the category is not an opportunity to 'pass the buck', to take the easy option or to relinquish responsibility, but to admit that sometimes there are no lessons that can be learnt.

In this chapter we will present a short case history to illustrate this category. In each of the settings (primary care, secondary care, the prison health care) that we have collected data, we have observed a small number of cases that were assigned to this outcome. The particular case study that we are going to present is drawn from one of the three prison health care teams that participated in our research (see chapter 7). The case describes a real-life incident, but as usual we have changed names, place names and some specific details so that we can maintain anonymity for the team and make our take home messages more accessible.

The chapter is divided into four sections including:

1. The team's history with SEA
2. The case presented
3. The solutions generated by the Team
4. Outcome categories

As before, we will conclude this, the final chapter by drawing out the main lessons that this team learnt when they reflected upon this particular case.

2   THE TEAM'S HISTORY WITH SEA

The health care team in this prison comprised a multi-disciplinary group of staff, including medical officers, nurses, and prison officers. SEA has a short history within the prison system and we were fortunate to be allowed to observe the development of the process in this, one of the three prisons where the technique was being piloted. The team in this particular prison had experienced a number of difficulties in terms of their relationships within the health care team itself (between health care and disciplinary staff) and between the health care unit staff and the staff of the wider prison. The team appeared to lack cohesion, with individuals sometimes appearing fraught and isolated.

SEA was instigated in this prison's Health Care Unit (HCU) by a senior management figure (a medical doctor) from within the Prison Service, who had developed an interest in the technique as a possible focus for improving quality and possibly for the then forthcoming clinical governance agenda. The Senior Medical Officer and the senior member of nursing staff at the observed HCU, whole-heartedly supported the introduction of SEA within the unit. However, the introduction of SEA was not welcomed by many of the HCU team, with some of the staff expressing their scepticism that this approach could ever be expected to work in the prison environment. A short introduction to the technique of SEA was presented to the group by one of the authors, in the form of a one-hour training session. Participants at the training session agreed to instigate SEA as a regular meeting.

The agenda for SEA tended to be set the day before the meeting, with the Chairman and the Senior Nurse agreeing the items for inclusion. Minutes of each meeting were recorded by the secretary, and distributed with the agenda to all participants prior to the subsequent meeting of the group. Agendas were flexible enough to accommodate discussion of 'hot topics' should it become necessary to include these.

The particular event for our case study was presented at the second SEA meeting of the health care team. Ten members of the HCU, including prison officers, nursing staff, medical officers, an occupational therapist, a pharmacist and a secretary attended the meeting. This particular meeting was chaired by one of the medical officers, although later in the process, chairmanship successfully rotated to a senior member of the nursing staff.

3   THE CASE PRESENTED

The case was presented by the occupational therapist ('Emma') to the rest of the group. The main points of the discussion are presented below:

> Emma described her frustration at the ongoing problems experienced by herself and her colleagues in the care of prisoners with mental health problems. She explained that a relatively high percentage of prison inmates had poor mental health, and some suffered from serious conditions. Emma described how the problem often became acute when 'sectionable' patients required admission to acute secondary care services outside the prison health care wing, but were refused admission by the NHS Hospitals on the grounds of their 'history'. Emma felt that the facilities at the HCU were totally inadequate for inmates with severe mental health problems, as the unit did not employ the services of a psychiatrist, psychologist or community psychiatric nurse. Emma concentrated on the circumstances of two particular patients to illustrate the difficulties experienced by people with mental health problems within the prison system. The group discussed the issue in depth, and drew on their wider experiences of shortages of specialist resources for this group of inmates.

Although this 'event' in fact consisted of a series of related experiences, Emma felt that it was appropriate to bring these to the SEA meeting as a 'significant event' because:

- It dealt with a long-standing, apparently insurmountable problem that seemed to some as a frustrating feature of prison HCU life,
- It highlighted a support need for the HCU staff,
- It highlighted the need for a change in policy across agencies,
- Discussion of the event provided an opportunity for catharsis and support.

4   THE SOLUTIONS GENERATED

Although members of the group agreed that this complex issue needed to be addressed, they felt that it was outside the powers of the HCU at this particular prison to change the way in which inmates with mental health problems were currently treated by secondary care services in the community. All team members agreed that this was a policy issue that required the involvement of the Home Office, Prison Service, the Department of Health and the Government. In the meantime, however, it was agreed that HCU staff should be better supported when they had to deal with these types of patients whom they felt really should be in receipt of specialist care.

5   OUTCOME CATEGORIES

The HCU team could not do any more to help inmates that required specialist mental health services in the community, and nothing further could be learnt from an ongoing discussion of the case. This case fitted into Pringle's category of 'Life's Like That'.

6   CONCLUSIONS

Whilst the HCU team were unable to reach any concrete solutions in this case, the SEA meeting did help them to reflect on a number of wider issues. These included:

- There was a consensus that teams do not appear to form naturally in prison HCUs; teamwork requires support and effort and SEA seemed one way of helping this process. It was considered important to use SEA to highlight examples of good team-working in action.

- Tensions and poor relationships appeared to exist between Health Care Officer staff and NHS trained staff and between Health Care Unit staff and the wider prison staff – there sometimes appeared to be a climate of mistrust. It was agreed that one of the ways of overcoming this was by discussing events in an open and supportive environment.

- Participants felt that there often appeared to be a lack of support at a senior managerial level within the HCU and the wider prison for change and the facilitation of change. It was reported that the collective efforts of the team could be harnessed to try to achieve this support.

- Because this team initially expressed considerable reluctance at attempting SEA, it was particularly important that the agenda of early meetings was 'managed' to provide opportunities for celebration as well as evidence of tangible outcomes – there was a need to engage team members and to encourage the feeling of achievement and empowerment.

- Leadership skills within the health care team appeared to be under-developed. SEA team members identified a training, development, and learning need for SEA chairmen. The role of the chairman should similarly be clarified and developed.

- The variable links with the NHS appeared to cause many problems for HCU staff, who often felt powerless to influence change. There was a recognition that in complex cases that it may be appropriate not to waste effort trying to change things that cannot be changed.

- There appeared to be a prevailing culture in the HCU that 'nothing can change', that problems are insurmountable. The SEA meetings highlighted the need to demonstrate changes however small, so that SEA could encourage ownership, and help to make staff feel more empowered.

References and bibliography

Essential web-site (including teaching material on PowerPoint)

http://latis.ex.ac.uk/sigevent/

Web-sites worth a visit

http://www.wisdomnet.co.uk/vconf.asp#cg
http://www.cgsupport.org
http://www.nap.edu
http://www.nas.edu

USEFUL BOOKS

Leadership and the New Science. Margaret J Wheatley. Berrett-Koehler Publishers Inc. 1999.
The improvement guide: a practical approach to enhancing performance. Gerald J Langley et al. San Fransisco: Josse-Bass 1996.
The reflective practitioner. Schon D. London: Temple Smith 1983.

BIBLIOGRAPHY

Allery, L.A., Owen, P.A. & Robling, M.R. (1997) Why general practitioners and consultants change their clinical practice: a critical incident study. *BMJ,* 314(7084), 870–4.
Andersson, B. & Nilsson, S. (1964) Studies in the reliability and validity of the critical incident technique. *Journal of Applied Psycholoy,* 20, 398–403.
Bailey, T. (1956) The critical incident technique in identifying behavioural criteria of professional nursing effectiveness. *Nursing Research,* 5, 52–64.

Baker, P. (1993) The Historical context of auditing and significant event auditing in particular. Paper presented at the National Conference on Significant Event Auditing, Castle Donnington.

Baker, R. (1995) Clinical audit in primary care: towards quality assurance. *BMJ*, 310, 413.

Benett, I. & Danczak, A. (1994) Terminal care: improving teamwork in primay care using Significant Event Analysis. *European Journal of Cancer Care*, 3, 54–57.

Berger, A. (1998) Why doesn't audit work. *BMJ*, 316, 875–6.

Berlin, A., Spencer, J., Bhopal, R. & Zwanenberg, T.V. (1992) Audits of deaths in general practice: pilot study of the critical incident technique. *Quality in Health Care*, 1, 231–235.

Bhasdale, A. (1998) The wrong diagnosis: identifying causes of potentially adverse events in general practice using incident monitoring. *Family Practice*, 15, 308–18.

Bhasdale, A.L, Miller G.C., Reid, S.E., Britt, H.C. Analysing potential harm in Australian general practice: an incident-monitoring study. *Med J Aust* 1998 Jul 20;169(2):73–6

Bradley, C.P. (1992) Turning anecdotes into data – the critical incident technique. *Family Practice*, 9(1), 98–103.

Bradley, C. (1992b) Uncomfortable prescribing decisions: a critical incident study. *BMJ*, 304, 294–6.

Brennan, Leape, L. & Laird, N. (1991) Incidence of adverse events and negligence in hospitalised patients. *New England Journal of Medicine*, 324, 370–6.

Brigley, S., Young, Y., Littlejohns, P. & McEwen, J. (1997) Continuing education for medical professionals: a reflective model. *Journal of Postgraduate Medicine*, 73, 2.3–26.

Britt, H. (1997) Collecting data on potentially harmful events: a method on monitoring incidents in general practice. *Family Practice*, 14, 101–6.

Britt, H., Miller, G.C., Steven, I.D., Howarth, G.C., Nicholson, P.A., Bhasdale, A.L., Norton, K.J. Collecting data on potentially harmful events: a method for monitoring incidents in general practice. *Family Pract* 1997;14(2):101–6

Brookfield, S. (1988) *Developing Critical Thinkers – Challenging Adults to explore alternative ways of thinking and acting*. San Francisco: Jossey-Bass.

Buckley, G. (1990) Clinically significant events. In M. Marinker (Ed.), *Medical Audit in General Practice*. London: BMJ.

Cantillon, P. & Jones, R. (1999) Does continuing medical education in general practice make a difference? *BMJ*, 318, 1276–1279.

Care, W. (1996) Identifying the Learning needs of Nurse Managers: application of the critical incident technique. *Journal of Nursing Staff Development*, 12, 27–30.

Cheek, J., O'Brien, B., Ballantyne, A. & Pincombe, J. (1997) Using critical incident technique to inform aged and extended care nursing. *West J Nurs Res*, 19(5), 667–82.

Clamp, C. (1980) Learning through incidents. *Nursing Times*, 76, 1755–58.

Clarke, B., James, C. & Kelly, J. (1996) Reflective practice: reviewing the issues and refocusing the debate. *International Journal of Nursing Studies*, 33, 171–180.

CMO. (1998) *A Review of Continuing Professional Development in General Practice.* London: Department of Health.

Crandall, S. (1993) How Expert Clinical Educators Teach What They Know. *The Journal of Continuing Education in the Health Profession*, 13, 85–98.

Crombie, D.L. & Fleming, D.M. (1988) *Practice Activity Analysis.* London: Royal College of General Practitioners.

Crombie, I. & Davis, H. (1990) Missing link in the audit cycle. *Quality Health Care*, 2, 47–8.

Crouch, S. (1991) Critical incident analysis. *Nursing*, 4(37), 30–1.

Curtis, P. (1974) Medical audit in general practice. *Journal of the Royal College of General Practitioners*, 24, 607–11.

Diamond, M. (1995) A critical incident study of general practice trainees in their basic general practice term. *The Medical Journal of Australia*, 162, 321–324.

Dixon, N. (1996) *Good practice in clinical audit. A summary of selected literature to support criteria for clinical audit.* London: National Centre for Clinical Audit.

DoH. (1989) Medical Audit. *NHS Review Working Paper 6.* London: HMSO.

DoH. (1990) Medical Audit in the Family Practitioner Services. *Health Circular (FP) (90)8.* London: HMSO.

DoH. (1998) *A First Class Service.* London: Department of Health.

DoH. (1998) *A review of continuing professional development in general practice.* London: Department of Health.

Donabedian, A. (1966) Evaluating the quality of medical care. *Millbank Memorial Fund Quarterly*, 44, 166–204.

Dunn, W. (1986) The critical incident technique: a brief guide. *Medical Teacher*, 22, 207–215.

Flanagan, J. C. (1954) The Critical Incident Technique. *Psychological Bulletin*, 51, 327–58.

Franks, V., Watts, M. & Fabricus, J. (1994) Interpersonal learning in groups: an investigation. *Journal of Advanced Nursing*, 20, 1162–1169.

Holmwood, C. (1996) How do general practice registrars learn from their clinical experience? *Australian Family Physician*, 26, 36–40.

Hopkins, A. (1991) Approaches to medical audit. *Journal of Epidemiology and Community Health*, 45, 1–3.

Howe, A. (1998) Can GPs audit their ability to detect psychological distress? One approach and some unresolved issues. *British Journal of General Practice*, 48, 899–902.

Hughes, J. & Humphries, C. (1990) *Medical Audit in General Practice: A Practicle Guide to the Literature*. London: King Edwards' Hospital Fund for London.

Irvine, D. (1990) Standards in general practice: the quality initiative revised. *British Journal of General Practice*, 40, 75–77.

Jones, R. (1992) Getting Better: Education and the health care team. *BMJ*, 305, 506–508.

Lemboke, P. (1967) Evaluation of Medical Audit. *JAMA*, 199, 543–600.

Lichstein, P. & Young, G. (1996) My most meaningful patient: reflective learning on a general medicine service. *Journal of General International Medicine*, 11, 406–9.

Love, C. (1996) Critical incidents and PREP – post registration education and practice. *Professional Nurse*, 11, 576–7.

Lyons, C. & Gumpert, R. (1990) Medical audit data: counting is not enough. *BMJ*, 300, 1563–6.

Marinker, M. (Ed.) (1990) *Principles*. London: MSD Foundation.

Marinker, M. (1990) Standards. In M. Marinker (Ed.), *Medical Audit and General Practice*. London: The MSD Foundation.

Marinker, M. (Ed.) (1992) *Clinically Significant Events*. London: MSD Foundation.

Marshall, C. (1993) Potential learning through critical incident analysis. *Br J Theatre Nurs*, 3(9), 23–5.

Maxwell, R. (1984) Quality assessment in health. *BMJ*, 288, 1470–2.

Minghella, E. & Benson, A. (1995) Developing reflective practice in mental health nursing through critical incident analysis. *J Adv Nurs*, 21(2), 205–13.

Newble, D. (1983) The critical incident technique: a new approach to the asssessment of clincal performance. *Medical Education*, 22, 401–403.

Norman, I., Redfern, S., Thomlin, D. & Oliver, S. (1992) Developing Flanagans' critical incident technique to elicit indicatiors of high and low quality nursing care from patients and their nurses. *Journal of Advanced Nursing*, 17, 590–600.

Orme, L. & Maggs, C. (1993) Decision-making in clinical practice: how do expert nurses, midwives and health visitors make decisions? *Nurse Education Today*, 13, 270–276.

Ovretveit J. (1999) A team quality improvement sequence for complex problems. *Quality in Health Care* 8:239–246.

Parker, D.L., Webb, J. & D'Souza, B. (1995) The value of critical incident analysis as an educational tool and its relationship to experiential learning. *Nurse Education Today*, 15(2), 111–6.

Pendleton, D., Schofield, T. & Marinker, M. (1986) *In Pursuit of Quality. Approaches to Performance Review in General Practice.* London: Royal College of General Practitioners.

Perry, L. (1997) Critical Incidents, crucial issues: insights into the working lives of registered nurses. *Journal of Clinical Nursing,* 6, 131–137.

Pringle, M. (1993) *Change and Teamwork in Primary Care.* London: BMJ Books.

Pringle, M., Bradley, C. & Carmichael, C. (1994) *A survey of attitudes to and experience of medical audit in general practice.*

Pringle, M. & Bradley, C. (1994) Significant event auditing: a users' guide. *Audit Trends,* 2, 70–73.

Pringle, M., Bradley, C.P., Carmichael, C.M., Wallis, H. & Moore, A. (1995) Significant event auditing. A study of the feasibility and potential of case-based auditing in primary medical care. *Occas. Pap. R. Coll. Gen. Pract.* (BPU)(70), i–viii, 1–71.

Pringle, M. (1998) Preventing ischaemic heart disease in one general practice: from one patient, through clinical audit, needs assessment, and commissioning into quality improvement. *BMJ,* 317, 1120–1123.

Pringle, M. (2000) Significant event auditing. In T. V. Zwanenburg & J. Harrison (Eds.), *Clinical Governance in Primary Care.* Oxford: Radcliffe Medical Press.

Qadir, N., Takrouri, M.S., Seraj, M.A., el-Dawlatly, A.A., al-Satli, R., al-Jasser, M.M. & Baaj, J. (1998) Critical incident reports. *Middle East J Anesthesiol,* 14(6), 425–32.

Ramsden, J. (1997) Objective analysis of a critical incident. *Nurs Times,* 93(34), 43–5.

RCGP. (1995) *Significant event auditing (Occasional paper 70)* Exeter: Royal College of General Practitioners.

Rich, A. & Parker, D. (1995) Reflection and critical incident analysis: ethical and moral implicataion of their use within nursing and midwifery education. *Journal of Advanced Nursing,* 22, 1050–7.

Robinson, L.A., Stacy, R., Spencer, J.A. & Bhopal, R.S. (1995) Use of facilitated case discussions for significant event auditing. *BMJ,* 311(7000), 315–8.

Robling, M., Kinnersley, P., Houston, H., Hourihan, M., Cohen, D. & Hale, J. (1998) An exploration of GPs' use of MRI: a critical incident study. *Fam Pract,* 15(3), 236–43.

Rolfe, G. (1997) Beyond expertise: theory, practice and the reflexsive practitioner. *Journal of Clinical Nursing,* 6, 93–97.

Rosenal, L. (1995) Exploring the Learner's World: Critical Incident Methodology. *The Journal of Continuing Education in Nursing,* 26, 115–118.

Scally, G. & Donaldson, L. (1998) Clinical governance and the drive for quality improvement in the new NHS in England. *BMJ,* 317, 61–5.

Schon, D. (1987) *Educating the Reflective Practitioner: Towards a new design for teaching and learning in the professions.* London: Jossey-Bass.

Scott, M. & Marinker, M. (1990) Small Group Work. In M. Marinker (Ed.), *Medical Audit in General Practice.* London: MSD Foundation.

Shaw, C. D. (1980) Aspects of audit 4. *British Medical Journal,* 280, 1443–5.

Sim, M., Kamien, M. & Diamond, M. (1996) From novice to proficent general practitioner:a critical incident study. *Australian Family Physician,* 25, 59–64.

Smith, A. & Russell, J. (1991) Using critical learning incidents in nurse education. *Nurse Education Today,* 11, 284–291.

Smith, A. & Russell, J. (1993) Critical Incident Technique:. In J. Reed & S. Proctor (Eds.), *Nurse education: A Reflective Approach.* London: Edward Arnold.

Stead J, Sweeney G, Westcott R. (2000) Significant Event Audit – a key tool for clinical governance. *Clinical Governance Bulletin,* 113–14.

Stead, J., Sweeney, G., Westcott, R. (2001) Significant event audit: worth bothering about? *Journal of Clinical Excellence,* 2(4), 197–198.

Stromberg, A., Brostrom, A., Dahlstrom, U. & Fridlund, B. (1999) Factors influencing patient compliance with therapeutic regimens in chronic heart failure: A critical incident technique analysis. *Heart Lung,* 28(5), 334–41.

Sweeney, G., Westcott, R., Stead, J. (2000) The benefits of significant event audit in primary care: a case study. *Journal of Clinical Governance,* 8:128–134.

Teasdale, K. (1996) Using personal profiles in reflective practice. *Professional Nurse,* 11, 323–4.

Vincent, C. (Ed.) (1995) *Clinical risk management.* London: BMJ Publications.

Vincent, C. (1997) Risk, safety, and the dark side of quality. Available: http://www.bmj.com/cgi/content/full/314/7097/1775 [1999, 23.12.99].

Vincent, C. (1998) Framework for analysing risk and safety in clinical medicine. *BMJ.* Available: http://www.bmj.com/cgi/content/full/316/7138/1154 [1999, 23.12.99].

Westcott, R., Sweeney, G. & Stead, J. (2000) Significant Event Audit in Practice: a preliminary study. *Family Practice,* 17(2), 173–179.

Woolsey, L. (1986) The critical incident technique: an innovative qualitative method of research. *Canadian Journal of Counselling,* 20, 242–254.